"*The Intuitive Eating Treatment Manual* by Blair Burnette is an essential, scientifically informed, and transdiagnostic guide for nutritional and mental health professionals. Effectively weaving the how-tos of delivering intuitive eating therapeutically and the important body of knowledge related to weight stigma and body image, this guide will become one of your most effective tools for working with clients who seek a better relationship with food and their bodies."

—**Catherine Cook-Cottone, PhD, C-IAYT**, licensed psychologist; certified yoga therapist; author; and professor at the University at Buffalo, State University of New York

"Health care professionals will discover Burnette's *The Intuitive Eating Treatment Manual* to be an indispensable leadership companion to *The Intuitive Eating Workbook*, whether you facilitate group or individual sessions. It's written in a friendly tone, complemented by useful worksheets and exercises. The manual offers practical suggestions for adjusting the length of intuitive eating sessions. Additionally, academics will value the included summary of research on intuitive eating studies conducted to date."

—**Evelyn Tribole, MS, RDN**, coauthor and cocreator of *Intuitive Eating*

"I have been waiting for this book! Burnette provides a resource that will be incredibly valuable to those of us working with individuals suffering from body image or eating concerns. Intuitive eating offers an antidote to dysfunctional cultural messaging about food, but the application of intuitive eating can be very challenging, especially for people with histories of disordered eating. Implementing the activities, measures, and instructions offered in *The Intuitive Eating Treatment Manual* will literally prove lifesaving for many!"

—**Charlotte Markey**, professor of psychology at Rutgers University, and author of *The Body Image Book* series

"I am filled with gratitude for Blair Burnette's enthusiasm and commitment to intuitive eating. Her focus on social justice aligns with intuitive eating values, and is a stepping stone toward removing structural and social barriers to eating intuitively. *The Intuitive Eating Treatment Manual* offers an effective guidebook for clinicians looking to help their clients embrace intuitive eating, increase their quality of life, and reduce their risk of developing an eating disorder."

—**Elyse Resch, MS, RDN, CEDS-S**, nutrition therapist, coauthor and cocreator of *Intuitive Eating*, and author of *The Intuitive Eating Workbook for Teens*

"In today's day and age, finding peace with our bodies and with food is a radical act, and one that has never been more necessary than now. Blair Burnette, an esteemed body image and intuitive eating researcher, provides a clear, evidence-based plan to guide clients on their path to a more positive body image and to a balanced, joyful relationship to food and eating."

—**Jessica M. Alleva**, assistant professor at Maastricht University, The Netherlands; and associate editor of the journal *Body Image*

"Burnette's timely and engaging guide invites readers to a cornucopia of evidence-based practical wisdom appealing to the palates of practitioners, scholars, and implementation scientists alike. It innovatively centers contemporary developments in the field from a trauma-informed, culturally humble, and socially just stance. This accessible volume amplifies topics not typically tackled in comparable manuals, appreciating the nuances surrounding food insecurity and flexibly adapting content to accommodate a diverse spectrum of pragmatic realities."

—**Jennifer B. Webb, PhD, RYT-200**, associate professor of psychological science and health psychology at UNC Charlotte, and associate editor of the journal *Body Image*

The Intuitive Eating Treatment Manual

An Essential Guide for
Nutrition and Mental Health Professionals

BLAIR BURNETTE, PHD

New Harbinger Publications, Inc.

Publisher's Note

This publication is designed to provide accurate and authoritative information in regard to the subject matter covered. It is sold with the understanding that the publisher is not engaged in rendering psychological, financial, legal, or other professional services. If expert assistance or counseling is needed, the services of a competent professional should be sought.

NEW HARBINGER PUBLICATIONS is a registered trademark of New Harbinger Publications, Inc.

New Harbinger Publications is an employee-owned company.

Copyright © 2024 by Blair Burnette
New Harbinger Publications, Inc.
5720 Shattuck Avenue
Oakland, CA 94609
www.newharbinger.com

All Rights Reserved

Cover design by Amy Daniel

Acquired by Ryan Buresh

Edited by Clancy Drake

Library of Congress Cataloging-in-Publication Data on file

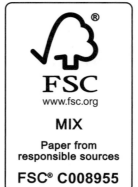

Printed in the United States of America

26	25	24								
10	9	8	7	6	5	4	3	2	1	First Printing

Contents

Foreword		v
Acknowledgments		vii
Introduction		1
Chapter 1	What Is Intuitive Eating?	7
Chapter 2	Working with the Client in Front of You	19
Chapter 3	Putting the Treatment into Practice	30
Chapter 4	Session 1: Ditching Dieting	45
Chapter 5	Session 2: Honoring Your Hunger	62
Chapter 6	Session 3: Finding Peace with Food	72
Chapter 7	Session 4: Challenging Thought Patterns	87
Chapter 8	Session 5: Fullness and Satisfaction	99
Chapter 9	Session 6: The Role of Emotions	113
Chapter 10	Session 7: Body Respect	124
Chapter 11	Session 8: Finding Joy in Movement	138
Chapter 12	Session 9: Gentle Nutrition	150
Chapter 13	Session 10: Celebrating Progress and Planning for the Future	166
Appendix		175
References		177
Index		189

Foreword

As clinicians, we want to remove our clients' symptoms of ill-being *and* move them toward well-being. Likewise, as clinical researchers, we want to devote resources toward studying interventions that alleviate distress *and* promote flourishing. Intuitive eating can facilitate these endeavors.

Several years ago, I was contacted by a graduate school mentor. Her clients had begun inquiring about intuitive eating and the possibility of integrating it within their treatment. She was intrigued and began reading about intuitive eating. She recognized my name within intuitive eating research and asked if I knew of a relevant clinical guide or manual. She wanted her treatment to be grounded in Tribole and Resch's ten principles rather than be swayed by media stereotypes or notions—some of which her clients had internalized (e.g., "intuitive eating is eating only when hungry"). She wanted to understand when timing was right to introduce each principle into treatment. She needed activities and help throughout this process.

Alas, I told her that there was no published guide or manual at the time.

You may be in a similar situation. Perhaps intuitive eating makes a lot of sense to you, and you are eager to incorporate it into your practice. Perhaps you are skeptical about intuitive eating, but you are open-minded to learning what it is about at your clients' request. Perhaps you want to study whether (and for whom) intuitive eating interventions are effective. You need a published manual.

There is now a published clinical manual (i.e., this one!), and it is phenomenal. *The Intuitive Eating Treatment Manual* is what you've been looking for.

Written by Dr. Blair Burnette, this manual is theoretically and empirically driven. You'll recognize concepts from therapy approaches such as acceptance and commitment therapy, cognitive behavioral therapy, and dialectical behavior therapy interwoven throughout its design. When delivered, it has been shown to improve intuitive eating, body image, and well-being among a diverse group of women with disordered eating.

Throughout this manual, intuitive eating is presented as a *flexible* approach to eating, with each of Tribole and Resch's ten principles represented within its own chapter. Client *nourishment* is top priority, including medical stability for clients with histories of eating disorders. It recognizes that intuitive eating is built on a foundation of *self-compassion* and *self-care*. It is an *inclusive* program that considers how dieting histories, trauma, eating disorders, food insecurity, neurodivergence, medical conditions, and other biopsychosocial forces can affect people's intuitive eating journey, and how clinicians can work to support intuitive eating among all individuals.

Wherever clients may lie on their readiness for each intuitive eating principle, this manual offers strategies for meeting them where they are. Multiple activities are provided to help clinicians individualize the treatment based on clients' concerns. Options for lengthening and shortening each principle, and for whom this tailoring may benefit, are articulated. Dr. Burnette troubleshoots and offers strategies to maximize client uptake of information. Clinicians are prepared for how they can support their clients as they navigate outside influences (e.g., others' comments on appearance, social media, busy lives). In short, this manual contains intuitive eating skills and activities geared for "real world" application and traversing intuitive eating amid the complexities of living.

Simply put, I cannot imagine a more impactful and well-designed intuitive eating treatment manual that will enable client progress *and* serve as a roadmap for continued testing, such as RCTs, to improve intuitive eating delivery to all.

And now I have the pleasure of emailing my mentor to tell her about this excellent manual to use with her clients in individual and group therapy.

—Tracy L. Tylka, PhD
Department of Psychology
The Ohio State University
Fellow, Academy for Eating Disorders
Editor, *Body Image: An International Journal of Research*

Acknowledgments

I am deeply grateful first and foremost to Evelyn Tribole and Elyse Resch for pioneering this work and blazing the trail. Evelyn, I am so grateful for your support and that you answered that initial, (over)eager email many years ago. This book wouldn't exist without you!

I have been fortunate to have many incredible mentors over the years. Special thanks to my graduate advisor, Suzanne Mazzeo, who let me run with my idea to conduct a randomized clinical trial as a graduate student. I had no idea this intervention would lay the foundation for my career and introduce me to so many wonderful people. Thank you to Tracy L. Tylka for putting intuitive eating on the research map and for inviting me into your work on the topic. I don't deserve my friends (cough, Sam, Mallory, Ted, Bill, cough) who have cheered me on and listened to my endless accounts of the trials and tribulations of writing a book. I appreciate my editors Ryan and Madison for their supportive feedback and bearing with me over the last year as I stressed about deadlines. And thank you to my parents—I know you don't totally understand what it is I do every day (as evidenced by my mom's cheerful calls just to say hi at 2 p.m. on a workday), but you're endlessly proud nonetheless. You always let me go boldly in the direction of what I wanted; if you hadn't nurtured that quality in me, this book would not be.

Finally, I am forever indebted to the many clients who shaped my thinking and the words within this book. It is the honor of my life that you have trusted me to walk alongside you as you seek peace in your relationships with food and body image.

Introduction

If you're a clinician, regardless of the populations you work with or your area of expertise, the topics of body image and eating likely come up. Unfortunately, these days it's challenging for *anyone* to feel at home in their body, experience peace with eating, *and* have dependable, sufficient access to a variety of nutritious and pleasurable foods. Poverty and food insecurity are long-standing structural inequities that have disproportionately and systematically affected certain groups, including Black and Brown people in the United States (Crimmins et al., 2004). There is increasing awareness that body image and eating-related disturbances cut across gender, race, ethnicity, culture, sexual orientation, age, body size, and socioeconomic status (Burke et al., 2023; Burnette, Luzier, et al., 2022; Cheng et al., 2019; Galmiche et al., 2019). Few people remain untouched.

People wanting help for these issues face an uphill battle. Weight stigma is pervasive and socially acceptable; appearance ideals are narrow and unattainable; and diet culture surrounds us with its endless rebrands of the same false hopes (Owen & Laurel-Seller, 2000; Puhl et al., 2015; Rodgers et al., 2021). Food lobbying and marketing powerfully shape our food system, and food insecurity remains a public health crisis that disproportionately affects marginalized groups (Coleman-Jensen et al., 2021; Hawkins & Panzera, 2021). Thus, having the tools to help your clients when the topics of body image and eating come up is *crucial*.

The inspiration for this guide developed in response to my own desperation to help the communities I served construct a sustainable way of relating to their bodies, food, and eating. During my graduate education, I became increasingly aware that different treatments were recommended based on one's body size and behaviors. Those in a thin body or engaging in restrictive eating or compulsive exercise were generally recommended to be more flexible with food, reintroduce previously feared foods, and accept their bodies. Those in larger bodies or engaging in binge eating were often prescribed rigid dietary and exercise guidelines, encouraged to self-monitor their weight or calorie intake, and lose weight. Given that disordered eating rates are often the highest among those at higher weights (e.g., Lipson & Sonneville, 2017; Sonneville & Lipson, 2018) and diagnostic crossover is common (Ackard et al., 2011), these differing approaches just didn't make sense to me.

Intuitive eating seemed promising to me as a transdiagnostic approach appropriate for the spectrum of eating-related concerns. Rather than asking people to follow externally prescribed rules that differ based on current symptoms and body size, intuitive eating encourages folks to follow their own internal wisdom and meet their needs in ways that work for them. Because disordered eating is often chronic and symptoms change over time, it seemed wise to not only try to prevent escalation to full-threshold eating disorders, but also provide people with new ways of relating to food and their bodies. I thought intuitive eating might *increase* well-being and health holistically, rather than just reducing pathology.

I reached out to Evelyn Tribole, who, with Elyse Resch, pioneered intuitive eating. I wanted to develop an intuitive eating intervention that followed their original ten-principle framework. Specifically, I wanted to test my hypothesis that intuitive eating could help people with *any* type of disordered eating in *any* body size. Evelyn was enthusiastic about my idea and offered training and guidance to help me launch my project. I recruited 71 college women who were engaging in disordered eating and at high risk of developing an eating disorder.[1] Participants were randomized to either a group condition or a guided self-help condition, and all attended weekly sessions that covered the same one or two principles weekly for eight weeks. I developed the intervention materials based on *The Intuitive Eating Workbook* (Tribole & Resch, 2017), adapting the content for a young-adult female audience with a range of eating concerns. Results of this pilot trial were striking. Disordered eating, eating disorder risk, body dissatisfaction, and weight-bias internalization all decreased and intuitive eating, body appreciation, and satisfaction-with-life all increased (Burnette & Mazzeo, 2020). What's more, the changes observed at the end of the intervention were maintained two months later. For example, prior to the intervention, participants reported an average of four to five binge episodes per month (about one per week), which is consistent with the binge frequency criteria of binge eating disorder. At the end of the intervention *and* two months later, participants reported just one binge episode per month on average (a 70-percent reduction)! Although these results were preliminary, they suggested that intuitive eating might not just reduce eating disorder risk, but also confer wider-ranging benefits.

Since then, I've continued to work with clients of all ages, genders, and diagnoses on intuitive eating, and I never cease to be amazed at how the principles resonate. Intuitive eating can be hard, but in my experience the greatest challenges come from external factors rather than internal ones. It's hard to listen to, trust, and honor your body amidst weight bias from healthcare providers, food insecurity, income inequality, cultural appearance ideals, and family pressure. Therefore, I focused my research program on the determinants and outcomes of intuitive eating, trying to understand its benefits, what makes it inaccessible for many, and how to promote it on a broader scale. I came to believe that the principles of intuitive eating can help so many people. Accordingly, I am committed to doing work that both equips people with tools to trust and honor their bodies *and* removes the structural and social barriers people encounter to eating intuitively.

Purpose of This Book

My hopes for this book are twofold. If you are a clinician, I want you to walk away with the knowledge and skills to help your clients reconstruct their relationships with their bodies, food, and eating. If you are a researcher, I want this guide to provide a blueprint for conducting intuitive eating interventions so we can add to the evidence base and understand for whom this intervention works, as well as when, how much, and why.

---

1 I excluded and referred out women who met criteria for anorexia or bulimia nervosa, or who otherwise endorsed symptoms that would necessitate more intensive care.

Goals of the Intervention

Intuitive eating can be used to address a wide range of body image– and eating-related concerns (we'll explore potential applications in Chapter 2). The specific goals of an intuitive eating intervention will vary depending on your client(s)! The overarching goal of intuitive eating is giving clients a new, sustainable way to approach food and to see their body. Rather than teaching people rules about how much, when, and what to eat, you're helping them learn to identify and meet their own physical *and* emotional needs. Instead of colluding with societal messages about appearance, you're helping your clients see their bodies as more than objects to be viewed.

A word of caution is appropriate here. Though the "body positivity" movement that has become mainstream in recent years has espoused a kind of self-acceptance, it has drawn increasingly vocal criticisms. One is that the movement whitewashes and oversimplifies the fat acceptance movement originally pioneered by Black and queer activists. Another is that many feel body positivity is simply unrealistic in current Western societies. In an ideal world, intuitive eating would be a step on a path toward body liberation and autonomy: that is (1) freedom from the social and structural oppression that deems certain bodies as more valuable, healthy, and desirable than others; and (2) ability to make decisions about one's own body. There are still dominant forces that communicate messages about which bodies are "best" and that restrict one's choices based on body size (e.g., doctors withholding surgery until weight loss is achieved). It's extremely challenging for people who exist in bodies deemed unacceptable or less worthy to consistently feel *positively* about their bodies. Increasingly, body *neutrality*—reducing or removing focus on appearance and cultivating appreciation for the functions of one's body—offers a viable, and more achievable, alternative. In this book, I offer exercises that promote body neutrality. My hope is that, with this intervention, you'll be helping clients feel at home in their bodies and find peace with food.

Who Is This Guide For?

This book is geared primarily toward clinicians (broadly defined) and clinical researchers. This includes nutritional professionals (dietitians, nutritionists) and mental health care providers (psychiatrists, psychologists, social workers, licensed counselors, marriage and family therapists). However, other professionals, such as physicians, advanced practice providers, nurses, university staff, teachers, and others may also use this guide to develop intuitive eating programming. For this intervention to be both scalable and widely used, people in a variety of contexts must be trained to deliver it (*not* just licensed professionals). It's inspiring to reflect that the eating disorder prevention program the Body Project is now regularly delivered by peer educators (Becker & Stice, 2017); with this standardized treatment manual, intuitive eating has the potential for a similar reach.

Because intuitive eating still runs so counter to mainstream messaging, you will need to have developed considerable familiarity with it before delivering this intervention, whatever your context. I hope this guide gives you the information you need to get started with your clients. If you're new to intuitive eating, I strongly suggest you read this manual in its entirety before using it with clients. If after reading this guide you still have questions or don't feel confident yet to deliver this intervention, there are many avenues for training. In the free online tools for this manual, which can be found at http://www.newharbinger.com/52540, I provide a list of resources to learn more about intuitive eating. More information about becoming a certified intuitive eating counselor is available at http://intuitiveeating.org.

At a minimum, anyone delivering this intervention should have sufficient training and experience to have developed expertise in body image and eating concerns. This is critically important: insufficient knowledge of body image and eating concerns risks iatrogenic harm. This is *especially* true if you are working with clients with eating disorders. Most ethics codes require that clinicians stay within their scope of practice. Because I don't have specialty training in substance use disorder, for instance, I refer clients to providers who are skilled in this area. Similarly, because I am not a licensed nutrition professional or a physician, I use a team-based approach for clients who need medical nutrition therapy or medical monitoring. Therefore, please ensure you have adequate training and supervision before treating clients for body image and eating concerns.

Finally, being weight inclusive is *central* to intuitive eating. Encouraging weight loss is *incompatible* with intuitive eating. This doesn't mean your clients won't come in hoping for weight loss. Many will! You can absolutely support them as they work toward developing new relationships with their bodies. Further, you can hold space for the desire for weight loss and validate where it comes from. It's not a mystery why people would wish to lose weight or why they would struggle to let go of pursuing weight loss. The social pressure to be thin is overwhelming.

This work will be very different for your clients in fat bodies than for those in thin bodies. I began this work bright-eyed and naïve, so enthusiastic about intuitive eating and the promise of food freedom and body acceptance for my clients. Reality soon came crashing in. I've now had many clients in larger bodies desperately seeking freedom from the constant struggle around food. We would work together to normalize their eating patterns, stop dieting, reintroduce foods, and begin seeing their bodies differently. However, any progress we made was fragile, and vulnerable to the myriad sources of weight discrimination they faced in their daily lives. Encounters with healthcare providers could be particularly perilous for my clients, as they received feedback that their health conditions were their fault and that—this is no exaggeration—they were *killing* themselves if they didn't lose weight. These appointments could wipe away any progress my clients made and send them back to the restrictive diets from which they were trying to heal.

Given the omnipresence of weight stigma and how easily it can derail intuitive eating progress, you need to be equipped to navigate these waters with your clients. Several of this book's free online tools will help you learn more about fat acceptance and body liberation. Most of us have some degree of internalized anti-fat bias (just as we have internalized racism, misogyny, and so on), because we were socialized in, and exist in, this world. It is imperative that you work to decrease your own biases and be mindful of how they may show up in your work with clients. In the session chapters, I will highlight areas specific to the principles and exercises therein where anti-fat bias could come up.

Who Is Intuitive Eating For?

Intuitive eating can be *transdiagnostic* and *inclusive,* meaning it can be adapted for a wide variety of eating and body image concerns.[2] Some clients may be dealing with emotional eating; others may be restricting their food; and others may be engaging in compulsive exercise. Many vacillate among these behaviors or engage in them concurrently. Regardless of their current specific behaviors, all clients will benefit from working to find adaptive ways to meet their physical and emotional needs.

In fact, I think intuitive eating is appropriate for *most* adults—even those who don't perceive that they "struggle" with eating. However, and importantly, intuitive eating will look different depending on clients' identities, contexts, and eating concerns. One client may be focusing on eating according to hunger and fullness cues, whereas another may be working to eat every three to four hours because internal cues are out of reach. The beauty of intuitive eating is that its ten principles give it an inherent flexibility. (Though intuitive eating is framed in the mainstream as a "hunger/fullness diet," I don't see it that way: hunger and fullness represent just two of the ten principles!)

The foundation of intuitive eating is self-compassion and self-care, and if I've learned anything from being a psychologist, it's that most people could benefit from more of both. We'll get into the nuances of how intuitive eating might look with various clients in Chapter 2.

Why Is This Book Just for Adults?

It's possible to use an intuitive eating–informed approach with children or adolescents. It's just more complicated. Children being treated for eating-related issues—like children generally—need to be scaffolded toward independence, and will require more structure early on as they gain autonomy in eating. Intuitive eating approaches with adolescents can be challenging, as these older children have *some* autonomy over their eating but likely not complete independence—and, of course, adolescents are still growing and maturing.

Many great resources are available on child feeding and working with adolescents. *How to Raise an Intuitive Eater*, a book written by two dietitians, helps guide parents toward fostering intuitive eating in their children (Brooks & Severson, 2022). For adolescents, Elyse Resch (2019) wrote an excellent self-help workbook called *The Intuitive Eating Workbook for Teens* that helps guide teenagers to building a non-diet, body positive relationship with food. The Full Bloom Project has a podcast and several guides focused on body-positive parenting.[3] The best approach for children and adolescents with eating disorders involves a multidisciplinary team (physician, dietitian, therapist) with expertise in treating pediatric eating disorders; and family-based treatment is often the first-line approach (Academy for Eating Disorders, 2020). Because children and

---

2   Throughout this book, I'll refer to any body image–related issues as "body image concerns." I view this term as more inclusive than "body dissatisfaction," as one may experience body image–related distress that is not "dissatisfaction," specifically.

3   See https://www.fullbloomproject.com.

adolescents require special considerations and expertise, this book is geared toward working with adults.

Summing It Up

I hope that at this point you understand the inspiration for and purpose of this book, and the importance of embracing flexibility, inclusivity, and sensitivity when working with the model. In the next chapter, we'll explore intuitive eating itself, including what it is and what research tells us about its benefits and what makes it possible.

CHAPTER 1

What Is Intuitive Eating?

If you're completely new to intuitive eating, please pause and seek out the formative texts written by Evelyn Tribole and Elyse Resch (Tribole & Resch, 2017; 2020). Their websites and social media feeds also have a wealth of information to deepen your learning. Everything in this book builds upon the foundation they created.

Tribole and Resch developed intuitive eating in response to their observations that the typical weight management paradigm in which they were trained simply was not working. Their patients left their offices hopeful, perhaps initially sticking to their meal plans and maybe even experiencing changes in their weight. However, almost invariably, they would begin to struggle to follow their plans, their weight would plateau or increase, and they would feel defeated and ashamed. It seemed clear to Tribole and Resch that their patients weren't failing at the diets: the diets were failing their patients.

What seemed much more reasonable and sustainable to them was to help their patients get back in touch with their bodies' own internal wisdom. The human body has processes designed to regulate its sleeping, breathing, evacuation, and feeding. When we need to use the restroom (provided one is nearby and we're not in a timed exam or the like), we go. Although many of us are not able to sleep exactly when and how much we need, we rarely question whether the overwhelming tiredness we're experiencing is due to a genuine need for sleep. Yet over time, our relationship with our biological hunger and fullness cues becomes fraught. We may begin to feel ashamed of our hunger, question whether it's real, push it away, or even lose the ability to detect it at all. Fullness may become associated with eating *past* fullness, which may evoke feelings of shame, and lead to trying to avoid fullness. Or we may become so accustomed to eating beyond fullness that we're unsure what comfortable fullness really feels like. It's no surprise that people get disconnected from their internal cues.

From an early age, all of us are bombarded with messages telling us we need rules and guidelines to regulate our eating; these are especially punitive and shaming for folks in larger bodies. Our hunger and fullness cues may seem more like nuisances than helpful guides. Our disconnection from our bodies' cues may be further compounded if we have experienced food insecurity, trauma, oppression, coercive feeding, or certain medical conditions.

Tribole and Resch believed that a focus on helping patients get back in touch with their physical and emotional needs, rather than on following external rules, would be much more accessible and sustainable. Thus, intuitive eating, with its ten interlocking principles, was born. Although you'll likely be working with your clients to progress through these principles one by one, they build on and inform each other, together creating a synergy. Tribole and Resch laid out intuitive eating comprehensively in both their book and their workbook; I will provide a more concise overview of each intuitive eating principle now, and we'll dive much deeper later, in the session chapters (chapters 4 through 13).

The Ten Principles

The first principle is **Reject Diet Culture**. Diet culture tells us that we need rules about the frequency, timing, and amount of food and exercise, either because we cannot trust our own body, or we need to change how our body looks. Note that I am not referring to dietary rules that are medically necessary or are undertaken for religious or ethical reasons. Diets are typically rigid and are very difficult to sustain over the long term. Because eating "well" is seen as morally superior, breaking rules can evoke feelings of shame. These days, diets often masquerade as "wellness" or a "lifestyle," and may brand themselves as "flexible." One major diet company promotes itself as flexible because you're able to eat whatever you want—provided you stay within your points for the day.

Essentially, dieting and intuitive eating are incompatible. If a person remains tempted by the false hopes of dieting, they're less likely to remain patient in their intuitive eating journey. After all, each new diet promises health, acceptance, and worthiness; most promise these benefits are *quickly* achievable and sustainable. Although most diets make these and other false claims, the data are clear: most people will struggle to sustain diets or weight loss in the long term (Mann et al., 2007; Nordmo et al., 2020). Further, chronic dieting and weight cycling are harmful to one's health (Tomiyama, 2014; Tomiyama et al., 2010).

Younger people are often less familiar with the term "dieting," and may not recognize that keto, paleo, and intermittent fasting are actually diets. Yet, the latest wellness trends (e.g., clean eating) almost universally offer the same unsubstantiated or oversold health benefits that old-school diets do. Wherever your client is coming from, if they remain bought into diet or wellness culture, they'll likely struggle with intuitive eating. So the first step is to help them ditch diet culture by educating them about the harms of dieting, with particular focus on how dieting (overt or in disguise) has harmed *them*.

The second principle is **Honor Your Hunger**. Clients may have become entirely disconnected from their hunger cues. There are many reasons for this. Some may have a fairly narrow idea of what hunger (what I call "tummy hunger") feels like. For others, being attuned to their bodies may feel unsafe. Additionally, chronic or recurrent restriction can erode hunger cues, so clients who have had restrictive eating or experienced food insecurity may struggle to feel those cues. Working with this principle means helping your clients cultivate attunement to their hunger cues, learn the unique ways their bodies communicate hunger, and begin to incorporate hunger into their eating decisions when indicated. For folks who have diminished interoceptive awareness (awareness of internal cues), hunger may be less central to their intuitive eating in the short or even long term.

Principle three, **Make Peace with Food**, is about beginning to disconnect from non-medically necessary food rules. With this principle, you help your clients reintroduce feared or restricted foods and gain unconditional permission to eat when hungry. This principle works on dietary restraint theory, i.e., that when we deem a food off-limits (whether our restriction is mental or physical; Herman & Polivy, 1990), its reward value is increased and we can't habituate to it. You help your client gently begin to relax their rules around eating to break this cycle so that they see the problem was the restriction, not their eating!

The fourth principle, **Challenge the Food Police**, is closely related to making peace with food (principle three). Thus, I suggest combining principles three and four when treatment must be shortened. This principle is about helping your clients get curious about their deeply entrenched beliefs around food (aka the "food police"), including *where* these beliefs came from and whether they still fit. I love this principle, because it gives clients the chance to practice cognitive behavioral and acceptance and commitment strategies, including cognitive restructuring and thought defusion. These strategies help your client form and practice new ways of relating to food, eating, and their bodies.

Principle five, **Feel Your Fullness**, is about removing barriers to and reconnecting with comfortable fullness. As with hunger cues, many people feel disconnected from their fullness cues. This can happen for myriad reasons, including past experiences of food insecurity, chronic or recurrent restriction, and struggles with binge or emotional eating. Other things may get in the way of experiencing comfortable fullness, including distracted eating. Therefore, you help your client identify and address what is disrupting their experience of comfortable fullness. Again, if your client has diminished interoceptive awareness or early satiety, this principle may be less central to their intuitive eating.

One often-neglected aspect of eating, satisfaction, is integral to intuitive eating and is the subject of the sixth principle, **Discover the Satisfaction Factor**. Diets can leave people feeling unsatisfied, especially when whole categories of macronutrients (e.g., carbs) are restricted. This lack of satisfaction means that people may be physically full, but still feel the urge to eat. Generally, eating meals and snacks that are balanced across macronutrients (carbohydrates, proteins, fats) and enjoyable (this is key!) helps promote satisfaction. When treatment must be shortened, this principle can be rolled into principle five, Feel Your Fullness. When time permits, satisfaction merits further exploration, as it can be an elusive concept to grasp.

The next couple of principles may prove more challenging for some clients, so extra time spent on them may be warranted. The seventh principle is **Cope with Your Emotions with Kindness**. It's about finding ways to meet emotional needs without using maladaptive eating or exercise behaviors. It's crucial that clients make strong progress toward rejecting the dieting mentality (principle one) before they start working with this principle. Undernourishment or a deprivation mindset can lead to eating that *feels* out of control or emotional. It's also helpful if your client is able to distinguish signs of biological hunger from an underlying emotional need (e.g., comfort). The work of this principle is learning to identify emotions and then match these with an adaptive coping strategy. For instance, one may seek methods beyond eating to self-soothe when feeling sad, or may find forms of empowerment that provide structure and safety and do not involve turning to restriction or overexercise. Intuitive eating also recognizes that *everyone* eats in response to emotions sometimes. Therefore, we want our clients to have several tools to choose from so that any emotional eating is done with intention and awareness (e.g., a celebratory dinner or dessert with loved ones). This principle will look a little different for clients with lower interoceptive sensitivity or alexithymia (difficulty identifying and describing emotions). Ensuring adequate nourishment via other strategies (e.g., eating every three to four waking hours) will help, and emotions can provide insight into physical needs (e.g., irritability signaling hunger).

Similarly challenging is the eighth principle, **Respect Your Body**. In our culture, accepting the body we are born with can feel impossible or like an act of radical resistance. With this principle, we try to help our clients see that bodies naturally exist in many shapes and sizes. When we try to fit them into a weight or shape they're not meant to be, it's not only futile, but it robs us of precious time and resources that could be spent in other, more meaningful ways. Clients don't necessarily have to love the *look* of their bodies (de-investment in appearance is likely a good thing!), but they *can* move toward treating their bodies with kindness regardless. We can help clients generate appreciation for what their bodies do (without reinforcing ableism), rather than how well they align with whatever the current appearance ideals happen to be.

The ninth principle is **Movement—Feel the Difference**. Our culture programs us to view exercise narrowly. Indeed, I lean away from even using the word "exercise" because it calls to mind grueling, repetitive activities. For some clients, repetitive cardio or gym-based activities may be accessible and feel great, while for others, those activities may be inaccessible or unpleasant. Gyms also don't feel like safe spaces for many people. Therefore, this principle is about expanding your clients' concept of movement, exploring which forms are accessible to and feel good for them—which may change depending on the day.

The tenth principle is **Honor Your Health—Gentle Nutrition**. This principle involves challenging work for many. When I explain gentle nutrition to people, I usually say it's about learning to notice how different foods make you feel in your body, and incorporating that knowledge into your eating decisions. I've found it's easy for folks to get rigid about this principle, especially if they still have a lingering diet mentality. If such a person eats bread and later feels tired, they may assign bread to the "bad" category. This categorizing ignores that eating choices are highly contextual. If a nurse knows they are about to work a twelve-hour shift and won't have a break for the first six hours, choosing foods that provide energy and lasting satisfaction would be a way to practice gentle nutrition. Similarly, if someone notices they're hungry an hour before they're meeting friends for dinner, eating something that provides a quick burst of energy (e.g., a granola bar) lets them respond to hunger without leaving them too full to enjoy dinner. Teaching flexibility and attention to context are key in working with this principle. Additionally, it's crucial that your client has worked on ditching the dieting mentality (principle one) so they can feel more sure their motivations are coming from a desire for genuine health and well-being and not from what they've been programmed to believe is "good" or "right."

How I Conceptualize Intuitive Eating

My understanding and conceptualization of intuitive eating have evolved over time through my own research and work with clients, my study of the critical discourse surrounding intuitive eating, and my observations of mainstream and social media portrayals of intuitive eating. Mainstream media often misrepresent or oversimplify intuitive eating, fostering misconceptions—intuitive eating is painted as either a free-for-all, "eat whatever you want whenever you want" approach *or* as a "hunger/fullness" diet, where a person pays attention mostly to principle two and principle five, Honor Your Hunger and Feel Your Fullness. In my view, intuitive eating is increasingly viewed as the latter.

Both portrayals wash away intuitive eating's nuance and flexibility. An overemphasis on hunger and fullness cues means intuitive eating may be an approach only accessible to those who are neurotypical and those with the most privilege. A recent criticism of intuitive eating is that encouraging a person to notice, trust, and honor their internal cues makes the assumption of safety and ignores that many people have learned to overlook or dismiss their cues in order to survive (Castle & Aphramor, 2022).

Instead, I frame intuitive eating as being about meeting one's needs within one's own context. This may look like learning to notice, trust, and honor one's internal cues. It may also look like eating according to a schedule to maintain recovery, or eating when food is available when experiencing food insecurity. It may look like eating now even though you're not hungry because you won't have a break for many hours, or like using distractions to get through a meal because being in touch with your signals while eating is unsafe. I don't believe eating according to hunger and fullness is a requirement for intuitive eating. However, as I mentioned in the introduction, it would be naïve and obtuse to suggest that intuitive eating is accessible to everyone. It simply isn't, and my research shows that (Burnette, Burt & Klump 2023; Burnette, Hazzard, Larson, et al., 2023). Therefore, I view it as imperative that I not only operate at the individual level to help people eat more intuitively, but also work to dismantle the systems and structures that prevent access to intuitive eating.

The Evidence Base for Intuitive Eating

The first edition of Tribole and Resch's *Intuitive Eating* was published in 1995. Since then, research on intuitive eating has proliferated, especially in the last decade. Although much of the research to date has been cross-sectional, there is also a growing body of promising longitudinal work suggesting intuitive eating confers long-term and wide-ranging benefits. The strongest evidence base is for intuitive eating's associations with psychological health and health-promoting behaviors. There is promising emerging research linking intuitive eating to physical health, but that area is still preliminary. Some researchers have also looked at how intuitive eating relates to eating patterns and dietary quality, though I suggest caution when interpreting those findings. Finally, the generalizability of the evidence base for intuitive eating has been severely limited by the reliance on white, female populations and the underrepresentation of all other groups. There is some emerging data (much of it from the University of Minnesota, where I completed my postdoctoral fellowship) with a large, population-based sample of young people diverse across race, ethnicity, and socioeconomic status and, to some degree, gender. So we are slowly beginning to understand factors that contribute to and emerge from intuitive eating in more diverse samples.

Regarding intervention research, it is crucial to note that most intuitive eating interventions to date have *not* used the ten-principle framework as outlined by Tribole and Resch. Rather, many interventions that claim to be or are categorized as "intuitive eating" are actually either mindful eating, Health at Every Size (Bacon et al., 2005), an abbreviated version of intuitive eating (e.g., not covering all ten principles, or only focusing on hunger and fullness), or include intuitive eating elements alongside content that is decidedly *not* aligned with intuitive eating (e.g., encouraging eating according to the food pyramid, or including a focus on weight loss). However, evidence suggests that *true* intuitive eating interventions (those following the ten-principle framework) may not only decrease eating disorder risk and other negative outcomes, but might also yield wider-ranging benefits (e.g., increased satisfaction with life). Below, I'll briefly outline the existing evidence base for intuitive eating and point out gaps and future directions.

Models of Intuitive Eating

What helps someone become an intuitive eater? What makes it harder? When researchers are trying to understand the factors that contribute to an outcome of interest (in this case, intuitive eating), they often create a conceptual model. The existing conceptual models of intuitive eating directly informed the creation of the intervention in this manual. Understanding what makes intuitive eating easier and harder will help you help your clients.

Avalos and Tylka (2006) pioneered the first research model of intuitive eating, known as the acceptance model. This model theorizes that when close people in your life accept you for who you are, you experience less pressure to try to change your body. Unconditional acceptance makes it easier to appreciate your body for what it does, not just how it looks, and makes it easier to tune in to its cues. When you appreciate your body, you're more likely to want to treat it with kindness and honor its cues. Alternatively, someone whose loved ones judge or criticize their body is going to have a harder time accepting their body. When you perceive that people in your life think your body needs to change, you'll feel more pressure to diet. And, as we know, dieting makes intuitive eating basically impossible. When you're following rules about how much, when, and what to eat, you're not listening to and honoring your body's needs.

Augustus-Horvath and Tylka (2011) revised their acceptance model, adding perceived social support and resistance to self-objectification as key variables that foster intuitive eating. This revised model adds nuance to the previous iteration. Basically, when you feel others accept your body, you're less likely to think about how your body is perceived by others (i.e., less likely to see your body as an object to be viewed). And, as theorized in the original model, you're more likely to be able to eat intuitively when you're less focused on trying to change how your body looks.

Ultimately, the acceptance models tell us that perceived social support, especially feeling like your loved ones accept your body as it is, is incredibly important for fostering intuitive eating. The reverse is also true: lack of perceived social support makes intuitive eating more difficult. Because social support is so crucial, I offer tips for fostering it throughout this manual. I also provide exercises to help clients respond to and deal with *negative* social influence, such as loved ones who comment on their body or their eating.

Beyond the acceptance models, research into factors that contribute to intuitive eating is relatively nascent. However, there is valid mainstream criticism that intuitive eating is a privileged approach, less accessible for those experiencing disproportionate systemic inequities. For instance, "eating a variety of nutritious foods when hungry" assumes these foods are available and affordable. Similarly, body acceptance is a much easier task when you exist in a body that is not stigmatized. Until recently we have lacked data identifying populations for whom intuitive eating is accessible, and understanding why. My own current research focuses on the social determinants of intuitive eating, with the aim of developing a socioecological model of intuitive eating, integrating research within a US-based sample that is diverse across race, ethnicity, gender, and socioeconomic status. In this work, my colleagues and I have found that parental coercive feeding strategies (i.e., restrictive feeding and pressure to eat), parental weight concerns, food insecurity, and lower socioeconomic status are all associated with lower intuitive eating among a diverse, population-based sample (Burnette, Hazzard, et al., 2022; Burnette, Hazzard, Larson, et al., 2023; Burnette, Hazzard, Linardon, et al., 2023). This model is intended to offer a path forward for research into intuitive eating's facilitators and barriers (beyond the micro level) so that we can ultimately remove systemic and social barriers and make intuitive eating accessible for all.

The Measurement of Intuitive Eating

Before we dive into the evidence, here's a brief summary of how intuitive eating is most often measured in research. There are two main scales that assess intuitive eating: the less-often-used 27-item intuitive eating scale developed in 2004 by Hawks et al. and the more common Intuitive Eating Scale-2 (IES-2) developed by Tylka and Kroon Van Diest (2013). (Of note, I am part of a group of researchers currently developing the IES-3, a revision of the IES-2.) Because the original IES and IES-2 are the most commonly used measures, I'll focus on them.

The IES-2 has four subscales that tap the following intuitive eating dimensions: (1) unconditional permission to eat when hungry (UPE), i.e., allowing oneself to eat when hungry no matter what; (2) eating for physical rather than emotional reasons (EPR), i.e., the degree to which one eats due to hunger and fullness and not due to emotions; (3) reliance on hunger and satiety cues (RHSC), which assess how much one trusts and honors one's internal cues; and (4) body–food choice congruence (BFCC), which measures the degree to which one matches one's food choices with their body's needs (e.g., incorporating how foods feel physically into eating decisions). The IES-2 has evidence of internal consistency (people tend to respond to the measure in reliable ways), validity (the measure truly captures intuitive eating and not another construct), and invariance across gender (the scale operates the same way across gender).

Intuitive Eating Research

Below I outline what we know about how intuitive eating relates to health behaviors, nutrition, psychological health, and physical health. Our most robust findings support that intuitive eaters often engage in health-promoting behaviors and have good psychological functioning and adaptive attitudes toward their body. Data on dietary quality is inconsistent and research on how intuitive eating relates to physical health markers is still preliminary.

PSYCHOLOGICAL HEALTH

Two reviews have evaluated the links between psychological health and intuitive eating. One (Bruce & Ricciardelli 2015), focused specifically on findings among adult women. This review yielded 24 cross-sectional studies that found robust associations between intuitive eating and lower disordered eating, more positive body image, and greater emotional functioning. Fewer studies in this review assessed the link between intuitive eating and other psychological correlates, meaning the evidence is less conclusive. However, these studies did find some evidence of intuitive eating's associations with greater self-esteem, self-compassion, life satisfaction, coping, social support, and lower thin-ideal internalization. Additionally, two studies found that intuitive eaters were less likely to exercise for appearance reasons. Although promising, this review revealed major gaps in the research: the overwhelming majority of participants in these intuitive eating studies were white, female university students (precluding generalizability), and longitudinal research was lacking (preventing the establishment of temporality).

A more recent meta-analysis, published in 2021 (Linardon et al., 2021), yielded 97 studies. The authors used sophisticated statistical techniques to evaluate associations between intuitive eating and 23 psychological correlates grouped into three categories: (1) eating behavior/body image disturbances, (2) positive body image and other adaptive factors, and (3) general psychopathology. Although most studies were cross-sectional, five were prospective and two were interventions. Further, samples were more racially, ethnically, and gender diverse than in the studies included in the 2015 review. Still, white women represented the majority of participants.

Consistent with the 2015 review, the authors found that intuitive eating was associated with less disordered eating (e.g., binge-purge behaviors, restraint, emotional eating), lower appearance ideal internalization, and more positive body image. Further, the evidence that intuitive eating is linked to self-compassion, self-esteem, social support, and well-being was stronger and more consistent. Finally, the authors found that intuitive eaters demonstrated greater interoceptive awareness, positive affect, and mindfulness and reported lower anxiety and depressive symptoms.

These authors also made the laudable decision to assess whether the associations between intuitive eating and psychological outcomes differed across sociodemographic characteristics. They found that the link between intuitive eating and shape/weight concerns was stronger for white participants and weaker for Asian and Asian American participants. Additionally, intuitive eating displayed a stronger negative association with depressive symptoms among older participants. Put another way, this suggests intuitive eating *may not* be as beneficial to body image among Asian participants and *may* be more beneficial for depressive symptoms among older adults. However, longitudinal research is needed to establish causality, disentangle whether these associations are directional or reciprocal, and evaluate mechanisms. For instance, it's possible that lower depression makes it easier to eat intuitively, but it's also plausible that intuitive eating helps one meet one's physical needs (e.g., nutrition), thereby improving mental health. Thus, although the research is promising, especially for disordered eating and body image, further longitudinal and intervention data are needed.

HEALTH BEHAVIORS AND NUTRITION

For intuitive eating to continue gaining traction as a viable health promotion framework, it's important to examine how it relates to both eating and broader health behaviors (e.g., sleep, physical activity) as well as dietary patterns.

Eating Behaviors Flexible dietary control, which includes behaviors like taking smaller servings, compensating with "healthier" foods if less nutritious foods were eaten recently, and controlling the types of food eaten, has long been viewed as a valuable health promotion strategy. However, both Linardon et al. (2017) and Tylka et al. (2015) found that flexible dietary control was often not so flexible. Rather, people who engaged in more "flexible" dietary control strategies were actually likely to display more *rigid* control over their eating. This rigidity appeared to account for the associations these authors found between "flexible" dietary control and greater body image concerns and disordered eating. Conversely, people who ate intuitively had higher body appreciation, which was associated with less disordered eating. My analysis of these findings suggests that "flexible" dietary control is ultimately still intentionally restrictive and is likely not so healthful after all; rather, intuitive eating might be a better health promotion framework to endorse in public health messaging.

One robust finding is that intuitive eating is *consistently* associated with less dieting and lower disordered eating in cross-sectional and longitudinal analyses (Christoph, Järvelä-Reijonen, et al., 2021; Denny et al., 2013; Hazzard et al., 2021; Linardon et al., 2020). My doctoral dissertation research supports this: an intuitive eating intervention resulted in a significant reduction in disordered eating (including a 70 percent decrease in binge eating) that was sustained two months after the intervention ended (Burnette & Mazzeo, 2020).

Given these findings, it seems intuitive eating might be particularly valuable as a secondary prevention strategy to prevent dieting and disordered eating from escalating into a full-threshold eating disorder.

Finally, in a cross-sectional study of middle adult women in New Zealand, intuitive eating was associated with a slower eating rate (Madden et al., 2012), and a recent study found that female intuitive eaters ate breakfast more frequently (Hazzard et al., 2022).

Dietary Quality I emphasize caution when interpreting research on the association between dietary quality and intuitive eating. Typically, this research looks at associations between someone's level of intuitive eating and their dietary patterns (e.g., number of fruit/vegetable servings; fiber, dairy, or fat intake; or frequency of fast or ultra-processed foods). That is, researchers are trying to get a sense of whether intuitive eating actually maps onto so-called "healthy" eating patterns. Understandably, for intuitive eating to be widely disseminated as a health promotion framework, people will want to know if it's actually leading to "healthier" intake. Yet to date, many of these analyses display a fundamental misunderstanding of intuitive eating: researchers often pull out a specific dimension of intuitive eating, like unconditional permission to eat when hungry, and assess how it's related to something like calorie intake. I think these analyses (and subsequent interpretations) can be misguided and misleading.

A recent systematic review evaluated the association between mindful or intuitive eating and dietary intake within the context of intervention studies (Grider et al., 2021). This review yielded five interventions labeled as intuitive eating. However, one specifically targeted weight loss; one was actually Health at Every Size; another was acceptance and commitment therapy; and one was a different weight-neutral program called HUGS (Health-focused, Understanding lifestyle, Group-supported, and Self-esteem building; Mensinger et al., 2016). Thus, only one of the included interventions actually followed the ten-principle intuitive eating framework as conceptualized by Tribole and Resch. Still, despite the scant available data, heterogeneous measures of dietary intake, and poor methodological quality of studies as rated by the investigators, the authors concluded intuitive eating does not influence energy intake or diet quality.

Another recent systematic review evaluated the associations between intuitive eating and diet quality, again within the context of intervention studies (Hensley-Hackett et al., 2022). This review included fourteen interventions that incorporated either mindful eating, Health at Every Size, intuitive eating, or an otherwise non-diet approach: again, the included studies were not restricted to interventions following the ten-principle intuitive eating framework. The authors found these interventions generally resulted in a maintenance of or improvement in diet quality (which was heterogeneously defined), though effects did not always differ between the active and control conditions.

Outside of intervention studies, the evidence on the association between intuitive eating and dietary patterns is mixed. Several studies have found associations between intuitive eating and fruit/vegetable intake (Barad et al., 2019; Christoph, Hazzard, et al., 2021; Jackson et al., 2022). Another recent study found that college women with the highest intuitive eating scores reported moderately "healthy" eating scores based on a 24-hour dietary recall (Belon et al., 2022). This is an important finding, as the group who scored the highest on the Healthy Eating Index also reported the highest levels of dieting, a behavior we *know* is associated with long-term problems (Crowther et al., 2013; Loth et al., 2014; Tomiyama et al., 2010). Indeed, eating nutritious foods in a moderate way would certainly align with intuitive eating. But being overly fixated on the nutrition content of food is likely not only inaccessible to many who lack access to a variety of nutritious foods, but also could be indicative of orthorexia symptomatology, i.e., a fixation on "clean" or "healthy" eating (Dunn & Bratman, 2016).

Finally, several studies (including many international epidemiological surveys) have assessed associations between specific intuitive eating domains (e.g., unconditional permission to eat) and dietary patterns. In a large-scale epidemiological study conducted in France, eating for physical rather than emotional reasons was associated with lower intake of foods high in fat and sugar among men and women, and lower dairy, meat, fish, and egg intake among women (Camilleri et al., 2016). Reliance on hunger and satiety cues was also associated with lower consumption of dairy, meat, fish, and eggs in men and women. Conversely, unconditional permission to eat when hungry was associated with lower fruit, vegetable, and grain consumption and higher overall energy intake. Jackson et al. (2022) similarly found that unconditional permission to eat was associated with higher sugar intake, whereas body–food choice congruence was associated with lower added sugar and higher vegetable and whole grain intake. Finally, Lopez et al. (2021) found that one's overall intuitive eating level was not associated with diet quality, but the dimensions of eating for physical reasons and body–food choice congruence were related to higher diet quality, whereas unconditional permission to eat and reliance on hunger and satiety cues were related to lower diet quality.

There are several reasons I suggest caution when interpreting associations between intuitive eating and diet "quality." One reason is that intuitive eating does not prescribe rigid rules about how much or what to eat. It recognizes that pleasure and satisfaction are two integral components of a positive relationship with food and eating. Moreover, intuitive eating is grounded in the theory that dietary restraint, whether cognitive or actual, is strongly related to binge and emotional eating. Thus, unconditional permission to eat any foods (beyond those that are restricted for medical, religious, or ethical reasons) is critical for decreasing the novelty and reward value that can often drive eating past fullness. Additionally, it may be misleading to evaluate associations between individual intuitive eating domains and dietary patterns. Intuitive eating is conceptualized as a staged approach. Unconditional permission to eat when hungry, without rigid or prescriptive rules about *what* to eat, is a crucial first step to habituating to previously off-limit foods. When one perceives a food is forbidden, one is more likely to have a "last supper" mentality, which makes it challenging to stop at fullness. So, as a person begins their intuitive eating journey, they may have high unconditional permission to eat as they habituate to previously feared foods. Because people often restrict foods considered "unhealthy," their dietary quality could appear lower during this phase. However, once they have made peace with food and recognize that previously forbidden foods are always an option, they can then begin to consider what foods taste *and* feel good, without that last supper mentality. At this point, diet variety and quality may change.

It's the *profile* of intuitive eating scores that can tell the whole story. For example, I conducted a study during graduate school in which I found that women with *high* reliance on hunger and satiety cues and body–food choice congruence but *low* unconditional permission to eat engaged in the *most* disordered eating and had the highest body dissatisfaction. This profile potentially reflects some degree of orthorexia, a rigid emphasis on eating "healthy" foods. Thus, looking at associations between individual subscale scores and dietary patterns means taking intuitive eating's dimensions out of context, which is likely to be misleading. Intuitive eating principles are interwoven and interdependent; they aren't meant to stand alone.

Physical Activity Research on the association between intuitive eating and physical activity is scant and inconsistent. A 2014 review found seven studies (four interventions, three observational) that assessed associations between intuitive eating and physical activity levels (Van Dyke & Drinkwater, 2014). However, only one of the four interventions followed the ten-principle intuitive eating framework; the other three were Health at Every Size programs. Of these seven studies, only one found a robust, sustained effect of the Health at Every Size intervention on physical activity levels. Thus, there are insufficient data to derive any sort of conclusion around how intuitive eating relates to actual physical activity engagement. Furthermore, simply assessing whether intuitive eaters engage in more frequent moderate-to-vigorous physical activity misses the point. The ninth principle of intuitive eating ("Movement—Feel the Difference") is about finding forms of movement that feel good in one's body, which will look different for everyone and will likely vary from day to day. Some will find that yoga and gardening are their favorite forms of movement; others may love endurance-based activities like running or cycling. Some days someone may feel like their body needs a high-intensity interval workout, and some days their body needs gentle yoga or a walk with a friend. Simply looking at activity *amounts* won't capture that nuance and may miss the bigger picture.

However, there *is* evidence that intuitive eating is linked to motivations for and attitudes toward physical activity. One study found that intuitive eaters are less likely to exercise for appearance-based reasons (Tylka & Homan, 2015)—such exercise is linked to disordered eating, body dissatisfaction, and other negative outcomes (Vartanian et al., 2012). Recently, I mentored a trainee, Emily Spain, on a project looking at the association between intuitive eating and attitudes toward physical activity. She found that intuitive eating was linked with greater physical activity self-efficacy and enjoyment among a racially, ethnically, and socioeconomically diverse sample of adolescents (Spain et al., working paper). This is encouraging, as enjoying activity and feeling empowered to be active can lead to more sustainable behaviors through the life course. She also found that adolescents who ate more intuitively spent more time doing a broad range of physical activities, including team-based sports, walking/running, gym-based activities, snow sports, martial arts, and more. However, there wasn't a significant association between intuitive eating and frequency of moderate-to-vigorous physical activity. This makes a lot of sense: intuitive eating involves finding forms of movement that are enjoyable and feel good in the body, which may sometimes get the heart pumping and may sometimes simply look like play.

PHYSICAL HEALTH

The evidence for intuitive eating's associations with physical health is relatively limited and inconclusive. There is some evidence that non-diet interventions can yield sustained improvements in cholesterol and blood pressure (Bacon et al., 2005; Hawley et al., 2008; Mensinger et al., 2016). However, other non-diet interventions had null effects (Van Dyke & Drinkwater, 2014). An older cross-sectional study of college women found that intuitive eating was associated with lower triglycerides, higher HDL cholesterol, and improved cardiovascular risk (Hawks et al., 2005). A more recent study found that higher intuitive eating during pregnancy predicted lower blood glucose postpartum (Quansah et al., 2019).

Much has been made of intuitive eating's consistent associations with lower body mass index (BMI). Indeed, numerous studies have even investigated whether intuitive eating could be a viable weight loss approach. Part of the issue with this research is it assumes that intuitive eating leads to lower BMI, without considering that lower BMI could make intuitive eating easier and more accessible. Indeed, Tylka, Calogero, and Mensinger (2019) conducted a study that provided support for the idea that the link between BMI and intuitive eating may be driven by thin privilege: those who are naturally in smaller bodies may have the privilege to eat more intuitively because they do not get the same level of messaging that their bodies are wrong or in need of control or modification.

Intuitive eating's evidence base keeps growing; new research is constantly being published. The evidence is pretty solid that people who eat more intuitively have better body image and self-esteem, are less likely to diet, and engage in far less disordered eating. Intuitive eaters also appear to have more adaptive reasons for engaging in movement, prioritizing its mental and physical health benefits over its role in changing their appearance. Some evidence suggests intuitive eaters engage in more health-promoting behaviors (e.g., less screen time, more sleep, slower eating). And a small but growing body of research suggests intuitive eating may confer physical health benefits.

Bringing It All Together

In this chapter, we covered intuitive eating's ten principles and its promising and growing research base! The principles are interlocking, flexible, and comprehensive, encompassing attuned eating, effective coping, body appreciation, mindful movement, and gentle nutrition. Research suggests that people who eat intuitively have a healthy self-esteem, appreciate their bodies, and engage in health-promoting behaviors. In the next chapter, we'll discuss how to work with the client in front of you—that is, what it looks like to collaborate with your client within an inclusive intuitive eating framework.

CHAPTER 2

Working with the Client in Front of You

Body image and eating concerns can affect almost anyone. In this chapter, I'll debunk common stereotypes, cover the array of concerns your clients may have (from body image disturbances to eating disorders), and provide in-depth guidance for working with clients who may need additional support around implementing intuitive eating (e.g., athletes). By the end of the chapter, you should feel more prepared to work with clients who are diverse in presenting concern, background, and identities!

Busting Stigma, Stereotypes, and Assumptions

Anyone can experience body image or eating concerns. For decades, the misconception that body image and eating concerns only affect thin, affluent, white girls and women pervaded mainstream discourse, treatment, and research. Scholars began contesting this assumption in the 1980s, providing compelling evidence that, not only do people across race, ethnicity, gender, and socioeconomic status experience eating concerns, but people not fitting the stereotype have unique and important risk factors (e.g., acculturation, discrimination) that can increase their susceptibility to disordered eating (Andersen & Hay, 1985; Iijima Hall, 1995; Root, 1990; Smolak & Striegel-Moore, 2004).

One reason body image and eating disorders became so closely associated with white women is that case studies involving white women informed the development of the original diagnostic criteria for eating disorders. In turn, because interventions are designed to target key symptoms and risk factors (those diagnostic criteria), our earliest and most-researched treatments were developed with white women in mind. Another reason that these stereotypes are so entrenched is that there are pervasive and enduring disparities in research enrollment, limiting our understanding of how eating concerns present across other groups. Accordingly, people not fitting the stereotype of whom eating disorders affect have been presumed to be protected.

We now have abundant evidence that these stereotypes are not only inaccurate, but also *extremely harmful*. Body image and eating concerns affect people across gender, sexual orientation, race, ethnicity, age, socioeconomic status, and weight status. Indeed, many marginalized groups have *heightened* risk, but are the least likely to seek, be referred to, and receive help for their concerns. There is fairly consistent evidence that people who identify as gay, bisexual, lesbian, queer, gender nonbinary, gender expansive, and transgender have higher rates of body image concerns and disordered eating than straight and cisgender people (Calzo et al., 2017;

Diemer et al., 2018; Hartman-Munick et al., 2021; Kamody et al., 2020; Meneguzzo et al., 2018). Men also experience body image and eating concerns, but they're less likely to recognize their own symptoms as disordered, seek treatment, or be identified by providers (Brown & Lavender, 2021; Strother et al., 2012). Accumulating research shows eating concerns are not limited to the affluent; rather, disordered eating appears to be increasing more rapidly in those at lower versus higher socioeconomic status, and food insecurity is a potent risk factor for eating disorders (Burnette, Burt, & Klump, 2023; Hazzard et al., 2020; Huryk et al., 2021).

We have limited data on eating concerns among middle-aged and older women and *none* on middle-aged and older men. However, there is evidence that women above age fifty are increasingly seeking treatment for new-onset, chronic, and recurrent eating disorders (Samuels et al., 2019). People at higher weights often have the highest rates of disordered eating (likely due in part to the pervasiveness of weight stigma and associated pressure to lose weight; Sonneville & Lipson, 2018), and are much more likely to be recommended weight loss treatment, which can cause serious harm (Hart et al., 2011). Finally, research looking at people with intersectional identities (e.g., LGBTQ+ people of color) is sorely lacking, but evidence suggests that individuals who occupy multiple marginalized social identities are at elevated risk for eating concerns (Burke et al., 2020; Panza et al., 2021).

Thus, it's crucial that you consider that anyone who comes to you for help may be struggling with body image or eating. Equally crucial is not making any assumptions about what *kind* of concerns your client has before they tell you. Checking your biases in an ongoing manner helps you not inadvertently cause your clients harm or disrupt trust and safety in the therapeutic relationship. Biases and assumptions can creep in in many ways. Because we are saturated with messages associating weight to behaviors and to health, and because stereotypes about whom eating disorders affect are so prevalent and enduring, we must engage in a continued, reflexive process to ensure we're not bringing our own implicit biases into the room in ways that will harm our clients.

Throughout this book, I'll integrate cultural and identity considerations that could affect how you work with your clients on intuitive eating's various principles. I'm bringing in my lived and clinical experience, and the wisdom of a diverse array of professionals and folks with lived experience. My hope is this manual will help you be inclusive and supportive of folks with diverse backgrounds, identities, and eating concerns. I urge you to continue your own work in understanding how interlocking systems of oppression affect your clients, and to practice within your competence areas. Education and consultation will be crucial when working with clients with unfamiliar backgrounds or presenting concerns.

Body Image Concerns

Body image concerns are *pervasive*. In our culture almost no one can "win." Almost none of us live in bodies that meet all the various cultural standards of attractiveness. The very few who do then likely learn their appearance is central to their worth and may experience lifelong pressure to continue meeting these (impossible) standards. It is therefore challenging for *anyone* to experience peace with and in their body. Nevertheless, some experience disproportionate barriers to body respect. People at higher weights receive ongoing messaging from myriad sources that their bodies are wrong and need changing. These messages come not just from media, but from family, friends, and medical professionals. Encouraging your fat[4] clients to respect and honor their bodies is a much different ask than for clients in thin bodies. Working with clients in higher-weight bodies will take additional consideration and care due to the weight stigma–saturated cultures in which we live.

For decades, body image research has focused on the thin ideal as the origin of discontent. However, the thin ideal is just *one* beauty ideal (and is *most* salient to white women). A curvy body ideal, with slim waist but larger breasts and hips, is more relevant to many Black and Latina women (Capodilupo, 2015; Hunter et al., 2020; Schooler & Daniels, 2014). Skin color, hair, and self-presentation are also often salient to body image among women of color. Women of color also experience pressure to look "put together," which generally translates to Eurocentric norms of professional hair, dress, and conduct. This pressure to conform to *both* Eurocentric beauty ideals and those from another culture (ideals often at odds) can generate conflict and distress.

Male-identifying individuals may experience pressure to obtain a muscular physique. Research shows that men who have high drive for muscularity are more likely to engage in disordered muscle-building behaviors like anabolic steroid use (Dryer et al., 2016; Lavender et al., 2017). Trans and gender-nonbinary individuals may experience gender dysphoria, which is often accompanied by body image–related distress.

Those who have experienced body-related changes as the result of medical conditions and treatments (e.g., chemotherapy, surgery) may also experience body image–related distress. Women with breast cancer, for instance, may struggle to reconnect with their feelings of femininity and desirability after appearance-altering surgery. Medical conditions that involve losing physical strength or sexual function may challenge men's conceptualizations of their own masculinity.

Ability status can have a profound impact on body image, especially within ableist societies where physical ability is assumed and bodily health is seen as a reflection of personal choices. Aging can cause body image–related distress as one's body diverges from societal appearance ideals.

Finally, working with someone who has experienced trauma, especially physical or sexual trauma, requires expertise and sensitivity. Trauma can disrupt a person's experience with and connection to their body.

It's important to consider that many folks live at various intersections of these identities. Those who carry multiple socially marginalized identities will likely experience disproportionate barriers to body respect, which requires recognition and consideration in treatment.

Intuitive eating can absolutely help folks who are navigating body image–related distress. All your clients will have differing relationships with their bodies, so how you approach body respect will differ based on their experiences and identities. For clients who have distress related to their shape or size, you should have education on anti-fat bias, including its consequences and

---

4 I'll occasionally use "fat" to describe people in larger bodies. "Fat" is a neutral descriptor, *not* a pejorative. Some people prefer to be called fat rather than other terms (e.g., people "of size"). Let your client guide the terminology used in session.

its racist origins.[5] For many clients, embracing intuitive eating and relinquishing the endless pursuit of weight loss will mean they remain in or recover into a higher weight (and thus a stigmatized) body. Glossing over or ignoring that fact won't be therapeutic for your client. If body image concerns are primary for your client, you may want to move the session on body image earlier or cover the content in two sessions so your client has more time to process and practice. This is especially true if the hesitation to relinquish dieting stems from a fear of weight gain or the desire for weight loss.

Chronic or Yo-Yo Dieting

Intuitive eating was originally developed with chronic dieters in mind. Evelyn Tribole and Elyse Resch created this anti-diet framework after working with clients who had tried diet after diet, emerging defeated—and more obsessed with eating—after each one (Tribole & Resch, 1995). Although their clients felt they were failing each time another diet didn't work, Tribole and Resch could see the truth: diets were failing their clients. They recognized that a deprivation mindset increases the novelty and reward value of foods so they're more enticing than ever. When someone's resolve almost inevitably falters, they're more likely to eat the forbidden foods with a last supper mentality: when you feel like this may be the last time you get to eat something, you're much more likely to eat it rapidly, without truly enjoying or savoring it, and often you'll eat it to the point of uncomfortable fullness. These "lapses" are often met with renewed (and even more extreme) attempts at dieting.

Younger generations may be less familiar with the term "diet," or may see it as something their mothers and grandmothers did—SlimFast, Jenny Craig, Atkins, or Weight Watchers. But dieting evolves with the times (it's a multibillion-dollar industry), and diets now masquerade as "wellness" or a "lifestyle," so younger generations may not realize that Whole 30, paleo, keto, macro-counting, detoxes, juice cleanses, Noom, and intermittent fasting are all just diets.

Because intuitive eating is an anti-diet framework developed in response to the futility of dieting, it's a logical fit for chronic dieters. However, folks will have different reactions to the notion of letting dieting go. For some, you'll see immediate relief wash over their faces. For others, there may be some hesitation or skepticism. Both are normal! The first sessions outlined in this manual are designed to introduce the concepts gently. You will encourage clients to approach what they are learning with curiosity, take what works, and leave the rest.

Disordered Eating and Eating Disorders

There is not one standard definition of disordered eating. Restrictive eating, binge eating, compensatory or compulsive exercise, self-induced vomiting, laxative abuse, diuretic misuse, diet pill use, disordered muscle-building behaviors (e.g., anabolic steroid use), and orthorexia all fall within common conceptualizations of disordered eating (Lavender et al., 2017; Striegel-Moore et

---

5 For reading about the racist origins of anti-fat bias, I *highly* recommend *Fearing the Black Body* by Sabrina Strings and *Belly of the Beast: The Politics of Anti-Fatness as Anti-Blackness* by Da'Shaun L. Harrison.

al., 1989). Restrictive behaviors can range from reducing portions to omitting certain foods, skipping meals, and fasting. Binge eating typically involves eating an objectively large amount of food (an objective binge) in a short amount of time. However, research shows there is little difference in the amount of distress and impairment that comes from an objective binge and a subjective binge (eating a small or moderate amount of food that one perceives as large; Mond et al., 2010). Instead, binge eating accompanied by a sense of loss of control appears to be a more salient clinical marker than the actual amount of food consumed (Colles et al., 2008).

Self-induced vomiting is the most well-known example of a compensatory or purging behavior. However, taking medications and supplements (including but not limited to laxatives, diuretics, diet pills, muscle-building supplements, anabolic steroids, and appetite suppressants) to counteract the effects of eating or to manipulate shape or weight are also compensatory and disordered. Exercise that is compensatory (to counteract the effects of eating), driven (to manipulate weight or shape), or compulsive (rigid, done when sick or injured, causing impairment to functioning) is generally considered disordered.

Finally, there is growing awareness of the disordered eating pattern known as orthorexia, which is an obsession with "clean" or "healthy" eating (Dunn & Bratman, 2016). Orthorexia is not yet included in the DSM, and some argue it is actually a manifestation of anorexia nervosa (Bhattacharya et al., 2022). Nevertheless, the rise in behaviors characteristic of orthorexia may be at least partially explained by the increasing ubiquity of social media and proliferation of wellness influencers and nutrition pseudoscience (Cheshire et al., 2020; Marks et al., 2020; Turner & Lefevre, 2017). The severity of these behaviors ranges; some are now basically normative (e.g., intermittent fasting) whereas others are consistent with a clinical eating disorder (e.g., extreme restriction).

Intuitive eating can be appropriate for folks engaging in disordered eating (especially considering how normative some of these behaviors are), with some important caveats. For my doctoral dissertation, I screened out women who met criteria for anorexia or bulimia nervosa and referred them to local eating disorder treatment services. I conducted further screening for any folks endorsing concerning levels of disordered eating to ensure suitability of the intervention. The reason for screening out folks with severe disordered eating is that intuitive eating is not an evidence-based treatment for eating disorders. This does *not* mean someone who is working toward being in or is in recovery from an eating disorder cannot ever practice intuitive eating. It also doesn't mean you can't scaffold someone toward intuitive eating during treatment. However, if in your clinical judgment a client's level of severity is high (whether or not it maps onto a specific DSM-5 diagnosis); if a client currently meets diagnostic criteria for anorexia, bulimia, or avoidant-restrictive food intake disorder (ARFID); or if a client is not medically stable, more intensive and targeted eating disorder treatments are indicated. If you're concerned in any way about the medical stability of a patient, then they need medical and nutritional stabilization before focusing on intuitive eating.

You may have noticed that in the preceding paragraph I did not advocate for screening out individuals with binge eating disorder (BED) or other specified feeding and eating disorders (OSFED). At mild to moderate levels of these disorders, low-intensity intuitive eating interventions *can* be appropriate. Some researchers recommend self-help (both guided and unguided) as a first-line treatment for mild to moderate BED in adults (Traviss-Turner, West &

Hill 2017).[6] Nevertheless, using intuitive eating as a primary intervention approach *may* be appropriate for individuals with BED or OSFED who are medically stable. I recommend further screening and medical evaluation for patients presenting with recurrent purging behaviors, especially self-induced vomiting or laxative or diuretic misuse, due to the risk of potentially serious medical complications.

In my experience, individuals with subclinical disordered eating, BED without medical complications, minimal impairment to social or emotional functioning, and no other contraindications (e.g., co-occurring substance use disorder) have responded well to intuitive eating. However, as detailed in Chapter 3, ongoing assessment and dialogue with your client is needed to ensure the intervention remains suitable and acceptable.

When Are Clients Ready?

There's no prevailing research to guide when clients in recovery from an eating disorder are ready to incorporate intuitive eating. So clinical judgment is crucial, as is the client's own informed consent. I spoke with several clinicians and researchers with extensive experience with disordered eating and eating disorders; all emphasized that clients with eating disorders should be receiving treatment at an outpatient level before moving toward intuitive eating. Clients at higher levels of care or otherwise undergoing medical, weight, or nutritional rehabilitation are not yet ready to focus on intuitive eating.

Brooke Bennett, PhD, a clinical psychologist and faculty member at Clemson University with many years of experience researching and treating disordered eating and eating disorders, described several markers that she perceives denote increasing independence with food and stability in recovery. These include when the client:

- Is medically stable and weight-restored[7]

- Is receiving treatment at an outpatient level

- Is demonstrating cognitive rehabilitation (i.e., fogginess has dissipated; "the lightbulb has turned on")

- Has decreased session frequency (e.g., going from every week to every other week)

- Is demonstrating sustained remission in disordered eating symptoms (e.g., consistently meeting a meal plan)

- Has an "exposure mindset," which Bennett described as a willingness to move toward fear (including willingness to tackle previously feared foods)

---

6   The utility and accuracy of the DSM-5 severity specifiers (i.e., mild, moderate, severe) are the topic of much debate (Dakanalis et al., 2017; Grilo et al., 2015).

7   See Steinberg et al. (2023) on the importance of accurate estimation of target body weight. Setting low target weights only encourages weight suppression and partial recovery. Clients may overshoot their target weights, which may be necessary for their full recovery and likely indicates the target weight was set too low.

- Has increased the variety of foods they regularly eat
- Has decreased cognitive rigidity (e.g., can adapt to unexpected changes in food-related plans with minimal to low anxiety and without compensatory behaviors)

Kelley Borton, PhD, a registered dietitian and faculty member at Oakland University, echoed these guidelines. Because intuitive eating is a flexible, nuanced, independent approach, it requires a firm footing in recovery. If clients are still undergoing weight restoration,[8] are medically unstable, or are displaying considerable rigidity around eating, they need more time and structure.

Working with clients with a current or past eating disorder may require special consideration. Whereas we often encourage eating without distraction in intuitive eating, incorporating distracting activities during meals *initially* can be helpful for these clients. However, since avoidance behaviors can often maintain eating disorder symptoms, unless it's contraindicated (e.g., by a history of complex trauma), I often incorporate graduated exposure exercises (both in vivo and between sessions) for patients engaging in food or situational avoidance. Working with clients with a history of ARFID may also warrant specialized treatment, especially if the client has never seen a provider for ARFID symptoms. Dr. Jennifer Thomas, a psychologist at Massachusetts General Hospital, specializes in the treatment of ARFID across the lifespan and has published a book for clinicians on cognitive behavioral therapy for ARFID (Thomas & Eddy, 2018) and collaborated with Kendra Becker and Kamryn Eddy on a self-help book for individuals called *The Picky Eater's Recovery Book: Avoidant/Restrictive Food Intake Disorder* (Thomas et al., 2021). I strongly urge you to seek out Dr. Thomas's work to learn more about evidence-based treatment for ARFID.

If you're considering incorporating intuitive eating into your work with your client, it's essential that they're on board. If a client indicates disinterest in intuitive eating or unwillingness to incorporate it, I recommend asking if they would be open to sharing their reasoning. Use zero pressure: they have every right to decline! If you notice they carry misconceptions about intuitive eating or don't see how it might fit for them, you can ask if they would be willing to hear more and tell them how you see it working for them. If clients are unwilling to discuss intuitive eating, respect that. They may wish to revisit the topic in the future, or they may know that intuitive eating isn't a fit for them now or maybe ever.

When a Client Isn't Ready

If a client isn't ready to discontinue their meal plan, you *can* still incorporate elements of intuitive eating. For instance, if a client is logging their meals and snacks, you can ask them to note their level of hunger before and after. Clients undergoing weight, nutritional, or medical rehabilitation *cannot* use their hunger/fullness cues to guide eating, as they're often diminished or entirely absent. However, noting their hunger/fullness can help them cultivate awareness of these signals and of how different foods may affect them. It can help clients learn *how* hunger and fullness show up in their bodies, which may be different than their expectations (e.g., expecting to feel

---

8   Clients *do not* have to be "underweight" (by BMI criteria) to still require weight restoration.

their stomach growling and instead feeling tired). When working with clients with eating disorders, I often use an app called Recovery Record. This app allows clients to log their meals/snacks, including timing, content (*not* nutritional information), associated emotions, and the use of any behaviors (e.g., restriction). Recovery Record helps clients get support with their meal plan and helps generate insight and motivation. It also enables you to individualize your clients' logs. I always turn on the option for my clients to log their hunger before and after meals as a way to practice interoceptive awareness.

Dr. Borton often incorporates intuitive eating principles not focused on hunger and fullness when working with clients in recovery. For instance, it may be useful to begin working on body respect with people who have high body image–related distress, given these concerns can motivate and maintain eating disorder symptoms. Finding peace with food and challenging thought patterns will likely be necessary as clients tackle feared foods and increase the variety of foods eaten. Essentially, it's possible and often helpful to begin working with some of intuitive eating's principles, even if a client still needs to follow a meal plan and is not yet ready to eat by following their hunger/fullness cues.

For people with lived experience of an eating disorder, intuitive eating may always look different than it does for those without such experience. Intuitive eating is about meeting one's needs. It is *not* the hunger/fullness diet, nor is it the anti-structure eating plan. People several years into solid recovery may still require structure in their eating to avoid slips or relapse. For these folks, eating three meals and several snacks every day at relatively consistent times (never skipping a meal or snack) helps them stay strong in recovery. I don't see these routines as being in opposition to intuitive eating, because consistency is what that person needs for their well-being. Within that structure, there are plenty of opportunities to integrate intuitive eating principles. Finding peace with food, eating satisfying foods, coping with emotions without using behaviors, mindful movement, and gentle nutrition could all be incorporated while eating according to hunger is de-emphasized.

Dietary Restrictions and Modifications

There are several legitimate, nondisordered reasons a client may have dietary restrictions, including but not limited to medical conditions (e.g., celiac disease), religious diets or fasts (e.g., kosher, Ramadan), and ethically informed choices (e.g., vegetarian/vegan). Again, I don't perceive intuitive eating as incompatible with these considerations, because intuitive eating doesn't require that people eat *all* foods.

Medically Necessary Modifications

If your client has medically necessary dietary restrictions or considerations and you're not a dietitian, I recommend you collaborate with a dietitian with expertise in both disordered eating and medical nutrition therapy to provide care, contingent on your client's insurance coverage and financial resources. If you don't have expertise, at a *minimum* you will need to seek consultation.

Meghan Cichy, RD, has been instrumental in creating weight-inclusive medical nutrition therapy handouts[9] for a variety of conditions from cancer, celiac disease, and kidney stones to migraines and polycystic ovarian syndrome (among others). These handouts can support your clients in navigating any medically necessary dietary modifications in a gentle, nondieting way. I've found that focusing on what to *add* has a more positive psychological impact than focusing on what to remove or reduce. Focusing on what one can't eat drives the deprivation mindset that can lead to obsessive food thoughts and binge eating.

If a client receives a diagnosis that necessitates dietary changes during your work with them, make space for processing grief and disappointment. It's a profound experience to lose access to pleasurable foods. And it can be challenging and perhaps fear-evoking to develop new patterns of eating. Certain medical conditions, such as hypertension, high cholesterol, and type-2 diabetes, may engender feelings of shame and stigma, because these conditions are often misattributed solely to health behaviors, despite their complex and multidimensional etiology. Educating clients on these conditions and helping to decrease this internalized stigma will be pivotal.

Dr. Borton believes that helping clients with medical conditions or financial situations that restrict food choices means that finding joy in eating is even more important. A former client of mine with newly diagnosed celiac disease found joy in discovering delicious gluten-free alternatives, such as a nondairy, gluten-free version of her favorite ice cream.

Finally, some medical conditions will blunt interoceptive cues or require additional energy needs. For instance, a person undergoing chemotherapy may have low appetite and high energy needs. They may have to engage in mechanical eating and find foods and beverages that cause less nausea but pack a nutritional punch—getting creative with adding fats and protein to smoothies and incorporating lots and lots of nut butter. Sometimes intuitive eating *is* mechanical eating, because that's what the body needs.

Working with Athletes

Working with athletes on intuitive eating requires special considerations. Athletes often have high and/or specific energy needs. Endurance athletes often work through their glycogen stores[10] during training, so these need to be replenished during and after hard efforts. The strain and stress athletes put on their bodies means they require proper nutrition and hydration to aid adequate recovery. Bodies are smart and resilient, so athletes may be able to get by on inadequate fuel or hydration in the short term. Over time, however, poor fueling and insufficient recovery will lead to performance decrements and potentially to injury or illness. Athletes may also have diminished hunger cues, meaning they won't always be able to rely on them to guide eating (Kawano et al., 2013).

Athletes have elevated risk for disordered eating and eating disorders (Chapman & Woodman, 2016; Greenleaf et al., 2009). Although this is especially true for athletes

---

9   You can find these online at https://haeshealthsheets.com/resources.

10 The body converts glucose from food into glycogen, which is stored in liver and muscles, and can be mobilized quickly for energy. So endurance athletes "carbo-load" before a big race and rely on sugar-based fuel during long efforts and competitions.

participating in sports emphasizing leanness (e.g., gymnastics, running), research shows that elevated disordered eating rates among athletes are not limited to these sports (Mancine et al., 2020). For instance, some sports require staying within a certain weight class and "making weight" for competitions (e.g., wrestling). Although the target weight may not be medically "low," the requisite weight range may be outside the athlete's set point, so reaching it can motivate disordered eating patterns (Satterfield & Stutts, 2021).

Athletes may receive disproportionate weight-related social pressure from society, their sports community, and coaches (Petrie & Greenleaf, 2007). It can be challenging to question the entrenched beliefs that a certain body composition is necessary for peak performance. However, attempting to fit one's body into a composition it was not designed to be in (e.g., losing weight to gain speed) will almost invariably have long-term consequences. Athletes attempting to lose weight may initially see a very short-term increase in performance. However, without adequate energy and recovery, the body will begin to break down. Relative energy deficiency in sport (RED-S) is a condition in which a caloric deficit results from an imbalance between energy intake and expenditure. RED-S affects athletes of all genders and is associated with endocrine issues (e.g., irregular or absent menses), dehydration, muscle cramps/weakness, anxiety, depression, difficulty concentrating, bradycardia, cold intolerance, and even stress fractures due to low bone density (Mountjoy et al., 2014).

Telling athletes to "eat more" without the right context is unlikely to be compelling or successful, particularly given the pressures they face. Providing athletes with information on *how* energy deficiency will ultimately hurt their performance (not to mention their psychological and physical health) is an important first step.

To learn more about working with athletes, I spoke with Christine Clark, a registered dietitian and board-certified specialist in sports dietetics. She mentioned that athletes are already deeply connected with their bodies because it's necessary for performance. However, because of the competitive pressures they face, their often busy schedules, their high energy needs, and the appetite-suppressing effects of exercise, they may be less attuned or less responsive to their bodies' fuel needs (Holtzman & Ackerman, 2019). Clark works to help athletes make connections between their fueling, performance, and overall well-being. She noted that this approach—wherein an athlete is essentially their own scientist—is much more successful and sustainable than her telling them what to do. If an athlete complains that they never feel good in their afternoon workouts, it may be helpful to walk through their typical intake leading up to workouts. Together, you can identify opportunities for change, such as rounding out breakfast with some carbs or adding a portable, energy-dense snack for class. As the athlete notices the benefits of adequate fueling, the changes are much more likely to stick.

If you're working with an athlete with disordered eating and you find they are unable to increase their intake or reduce their activity on their own, referral to more intensive treatment is likely warranted. When someone continues to exercise, restrict, or otherwise engage in maladaptive behaviors despite consequences such as injuries or illness, they may have a clinical eating disorder requiring treatment. Additionally, consulting with the athlete's coaches/training staff (if applicable) and an eating disorder–informed physician will be crucial. The physician can help monitor the athlete and ensure that return to sport is safe and that intuitive eating is appropriate.

Trauma

Although meditation and mindfulness-based approaches show promise for addressing myriad conditions, there is also literature on the potential of such approaches to cause harm for those with a trauma history (Duane et al., 2021; Van Dam et al., 2018). Responding to this concern, researchers are increasingly implementing a trauma-informed approach to mindfulness-based programs (Duane et al., 2021; Kelly, 2015). Trauma-informed approaches typically involve psychoeducation on trauma to give individuals a framework for understanding their symptoms and reactions with compassion, fostering safety within the therapeutic space, and teaching self-containment and self-regulation techniques to decrease reactivity to physiological and cognitive effects of trauma. Over time, the goal is to decrease the conditioned fear responses activated by the physiological symptoms that often accompany trauma. Without this trauma-informed approach, emphasizing mindful awareness and attunement may increase trauma symptoms without providing clients tools to address such responses. Unfortunately, without trauma-informed adaptations to intuitive eating interventions, we lack data on the best way to approach intuitive eating with clients who have trauma-related symptoms. If you have expertise in treating trauma or have experience in implementing trauma-informed care models, then you may be able to safely proceed by integrating your knowledge into the delivery of this intervention. However, if you do not have such training, I recommend referring your client to a trauma specialist when related symptoms are present.

Bringing It All Together

If your client is experiencing body image– or eating-related distress, there's a good chance intuitive eating can help. However, for clients who have a history of an eating disorder or trauma, or who have medical conditions that necessitate dietary changes, or who are athletes, intuitive eating may look different and will likely require multidisciplinary care. It's also OK if intuitive eating isn't right for a particular client right now due to more pressing challenges. They can always revisit it in the future.

CHAPTER 3

Putting the Treatment into Practice

This chapter is packed with information you'll need to get started working with intuitive eating with your clients. I'll discuss the intervention structure, theoretical underpinnings, ways to deliver the intervention (including considerations for group interventions), getting started (including intake and assessment), session structure, options for changing the intervention length, changing the session order, involving significant others, and considerations for research. Let's dive in!

Intervention Structure

The standard intuitive eating intervention format is ten sessions. You may have more or fewer sessions to work with, so I will also provide recommendations on how to cover the content in four, six, eight, and twelve sessions, and on spending more or less time on certain principles. At the end of each session chapter (Chapters 4 through 13), I offer more detailed information about how to shorten or lengthen each session, including what content can be omitted or expanded.

Weekly sessions are most typical, but you can increase the time between sessions if indicated. More time between sessions may offer clients additional opportunities for practice. However, *too* much time between sessions could lead to drift and compromise treatment progress. If you extend the time between sessions, consider including brief check-ins, which may help increase engagement by providing ongoing support and accountability.

Each session is designed to last approximately one hour. Our college student sample perceived 90-minute sessions as too long. Yet, longer sessions could be acceptable depending on the context. If your client or group is particularly chatty, you may struggle to stay within an hour and need to trim content or activities.

Each session contains a mix of psychoeducation and interactive activities, with between-session exercises provided to reinforce learning. Because intuitive eating runs so counter to mainstream messages about eating, considerable education is needed; interactive activities are necessary to balance out didactic portions, increase engagement, and reinforce concepts. Although many adults struggle to find time to incorporate "homework,"[11] such activities provide opportunities to practice new skills and to receive more feedback during the next session. Exercises in this manual are designed to fit within the realities of most adults' daily lives. Each week's exercises will focus on specific skills (e.g., increasing hunger awareness) that you can tailor

---
11 I try to avoid using the term "homework" with clients because it has associations with work that is tedious, required, and evaluated. We want exercises to be seen as opportunities for practice—not something that clients can pass or fail.

Putting the Treatment into Practice

to your client (e.g., minimizing distractions during dinner). Several between-session exercises are provided for most weeks, and you and your client(s) can pick and choose which make sense to prioritize.

Theoretical Framework

Theories are useful in developing an intervention because they give guidance on how to present the content, the types of exercises to include, interpersonal dynamics to watch out for, and specific topics to cover. Several theories informed the development of this intervention; I highlight why these theories are important to keep in mind as you are working with clients on intuitive eating.

Acceptance Model of Intuitive Eating

The acceptance model (Avalos & Tylka, 2006) states that being in an accepting social environment helps people eat more intuitively. Helping your client cultivate such an environment maximizes the intervention's effectiveness. In this intervention, you'll continuously provide and model unconditional acceptance and promote body appreciation. This might look like reframing negative body-related comments when they come up (e.g., "I hear you that you didn't feel good in the clothes you were wearing. Can we consider whether it's actually your body that's the problem, or maybe something else?"). Further, I encourage you to help connect your clients with communities and resources that are unconditionally accepting and, at minimum, body-neutral.[12] For instance, when clients are active on social media or listen to podcasts, I encourage them to take stock of whom they are following, unfollow accounts that are not intuitive eating–aligned, and seek out intuitive eating and body liberation content. You might consider curating a list of such accounts to distribute to your clients. If you're conducting groups or guided self-help, you may consider offering a moderated platform for participants to connect between and outside of sessions for friendship and support. I've had group members who engaged in mindful movement and did food habituation exercises together.

Theory of Psychological Reactance

This theory states that when individuals feel pressured, or perceive their autonomy is being threatened, they're likely to become reactive and act in opposition (Brehm, 1966). Therefore, throughout the intervention (*especially* in the beginning), encourage your clients to be open and curious, and honor their autonomy. I tell my clients to take what works and leave the rest, and I work to create a space where they feel comfortable discussing their reservations, skepticism, and disagreements.

---

[12] Body positivity may feel out of reach for your client, but if they connect with a community of people who celebrate their bodies beyond just appearance, then by all means cheer that on!

The first time I conducted an intuitive eating intervention, my co-leaders and I learned the salience of the theory of psychological reactance the hard way. In the first group session we led (ditching dieting), we were heavy-handed about the harms of dieting—and we unintentionally cultivated resistance and defensiveness. Participants couldn't yet see the nuances of intuitive eating, nor did they yet have a broader framework in which to situate what they were learning. So, what they heard was that being health-conscious is bad, that the rules they were following were wrong, and that we were threatening to take all of that away.

Cognitive Dissonance Theory

This theory states that people experience discomfort when there's a discrepancy between their beliefs and their actions (Festinger, 1957). This discomfort is so aversive that people are highly motivated to resolve the discrepancy. One of the most empirically supported eating disorder prevention programs, the Body Project, capitalizes on cognitive dissonance theory by using dissonance-generating exercises (Becker & Stice, 2017). Specifically, the Body Project attempts to reduce thin-ideal internalization through a series of exercises where participants discuss the costs of pursuing the thin ideal, role-play arguing against pursuit of the thin ideal, and engage in body activism (e.g., volunteer with advocacy organizations). The idea is that these activities will begin to change participants' beliefs about the value of pursuing the thin ideal, which will produce a dissonance between their values and their actions. Ideally, participants will attempt to resolve this discrepancy by changing their actions (e.g., stopping dieting) to align with their beliefs. Given the success of the Body Project, I've integrated some dissonance-based exercises in this manual to help clients reframe their beliefs about food, eating, and body image and motivate associated behavioral changes.

Social Comparison Theory

This theory is likely *most* relevant to group settings; it states that individuals evaluate themselves based on comparisons with others (Festinger, 1954). *Lateral comparisons*, or comparisons to others viewed as similar, are the most common, as they provide the most information on how one compares to various social norms and ideals (e.g., education, income, relationship status). People also make upward and downward comparisons, which serve to regulate self-esteem. *Upward comparisons*, made against someone viewed as "better" in some domain, generally decrease self-esteem. Social media is rife with opportunities for upward comparisons in the idealized images people post. These images promote sociocultural appearance norms, and because they are often heavily altered, it is easy to feel like you don't "measure up." *Downward comparisons* are those made against others viewed as worse off in some domain; for instance, comparing yourself to someone you view as less attractive or successful. Downward comparisons can (albeit temporarily) increase self-esteem. Social comparisons can also strongly influence group dynamics. As a facilitator, you'll need to be aware of how these comparisons could affect your group; I will detail this issue more when discussing group characteristics later in this chapter.

Intervention Modality

The intervention in this manual is designed to be delivered in individual or group formats, though I also provide tips for guided self-help. (You may get creative and think of other uses for this guide—if so, please contact me, I'd love to hear more!) Each session chapter contains considerations for delivering the session within a group, such as group dynamics that may arise. All session activities are written to be easily adapted for either individual or group formats.

Individual Sessions

The ten session chapters in this manual are geared toward individual, one-on-one sessions. The content for each session is designed to last 60 minutes; if you conduct 45- or 50-minute sessions, the content can be streamlined. If the number of sessions is limited due to insurance, financial, or other considerations, you may need to condense or streamline content. I will provide suggestions for how to do so along the way. I recommend conducting a thorough assessment prior to initiating treatment (see "Getting Started" later in this chapter): results can guide discussions with your client, and subsequent clinical decisions, about which content merits the most coverage for your client. For instance, if body image is your client's primary source of distress, you likely won't want to condense that content. If you can conduct *more* than ten sessions (and this seems clinically indicated), you can use assessment results and client progress to determine which content merits more time.

Group Sessions

Groups have many benefits, including cost-effectiveness, accessibility, normalization of shared experiences, validation, and feedback. Groups also come with challenges! Groups provide fewer opportunities for each participant to process how the content applies to them than individual formats. Group dynamics can also be challenging to navigate. Dominant members may speak frequently, reducing others' opportunity to speak. Though group members may have similarities and share specific concerns (e.g., members are female-identified young adults with binge eating), a group format is still less tailored than an individual format. Although our pilot trial was composed of all college women, the groups were still fairly heterogeneous in terms of other identities, and members presented with a range of eating and body image concerns. Thus, not all participants resonated with all material, an inevitability some participants cited as a limitation.

Because the nitty-gritty of conducting group therapy (e.g., structure, size, length, frequency, number of leaders, member homogeneity/heterogeneity) is outside the scope of this book, I encourage you to seek out further reading if it's new to you. That said, in this section, I'll provide considerations and suggestions specific to conducting intuitive eating groups. (e.g., discussing weight in a group where diverse body sizes are represented) and suggestions for adapting activities to a group format. The initial session will include time for introducing the program, group introductions, and co-creating group guidelines.

GROUP SIZE

I've been involved in group interventions with as few as two and as many as twelve participants. Ultimately, I think the sweet spot is somewhere between five and nine participants; this is reinforced in the literature (Burlingame et al., 2018). Group dynamics can become somewhat unpredictable with fewer than five participants, and absences are more noticeable and disruptive than in larger groups. However, once a group gets to ten members, it's challenging to get through the material and provide everyone a chance to share.

SINGLE-LED AND CO-LED GROUPS

I've conducted intuitive eating groups with one and two leaders. I recommend two leaders when possible; research shows co-led groups have advantages over single-led groups (Kivlighan Jr. et al., 2012). When our intuitive eating groups were co-led, leaders appreciated having someone else to fill in what they missed, offer an alternate perspective, and provide support for navigating challenging comments and interpersonal dynamics.

OPEN AND CLOSED GROUPS

Groups can be open (ongoing; members enter and exit at varying times) or closed (time-limited; all members enter and exit at the same time). I have only conducted closed intuitive eating groups; I perceived it was maximally beneficial, as group members were learning the content together. Nevertheless, we don't yet have data comparing the efficacy of intuitive eating groups conducted in open or closed formats. This manual is written with a closed, ten-week group in mind.

GROUP HETEROGENEITY OR HOMOGENEITY

When I conducted an intuitive eating pilot intervention, I was intentional about which characteristics my group participants would and would not share. The intervention's purpose was to evaluate whether intuitive eating was a viable transdiagnostic approach for disordered eating: would intuitive eating have comparable effects regardless of the *type* of disordered eating someone reported? Additionally, I was interested in demonstrating that intuitive eating was appropriate regardless of body size (i.e., we don't prescribe body modification to those in larger bodies while telling people in thinner bodies to accept their bodies). Finally, I wanted the intervention to be inclusive and *not* just for white women, as so many disordered-eating interventions have been. So participants in my intervention were heterogeneous in their presenting eating/body image concern and in their body size, race, ethnicity, socioeconomic status, and immigration status. However, I also wanted to target a group at particularly high risk for an eating disorder (female-identified university students engaging in disordered eating). Because participants were all female-identified students ages 18 to 25 at a large public university, they were homogenous in education level, developmental stage, geographic location, and gender.

Your group's goals and the extant literature should guide your decisions regarding group homogeneity or heterogeneity, and thus your recruitment strategy. Ultimately, we had success conducting groups with women who were heterogenous in presenting concern and body size. Women expressed that it was beneficial to hear from other members who had different struggles and life experiences. One potential concern with heterogeneous groups is that the dominant power dynamics that play out in broader society show up in the room. As a group facilitator, you'll need to be aware of and intervene on both subtle and obvious forms of discrimination, such as dominant groups taking up all the space or interrupting others, or other forms of discrimination (e.g., racist comments). Weight stigma is culturally determined and can also affect group dynamics. For example, Western cultures value and normalize behaviors like restriction or extreme exercise as disciplined and virtuous. Conversely, behaviors like binge eating or being sedentary are seen as lazy, unhealthy, and undisciplined. Similar dynamics play out between people in thin and fat bodies. Women who engage in restrictive behaviors or are in smaller bodies may feel more comfortable speaking up than women who are dealing with binge eating or are in larger bodies.

These potential dynamics are something you as a group leader must be vigilant for, as perceived lack of safety or security will affect attendance, retention, and intervention efficacy. I recommend that in the first session you explain that in group we do not see any behaviors or body sizes as better than others. In our groups, members were able to provide feedback via an anonymous online form, which helped us address dynamics that made members feel less safe.

Conducting groups with people with heterogeneous presenting concerns can be advantageous because it can help members see how each principle can be applied more broadly. Diagnostic crossover is common, and it can be useful for people to know how to apply intuitive eating if their struggles ever change (e.g., moving from restrictive to binge eating). However, a downside to such groups is there's less time to go into detail on how the principles apply to each person.

Guided Self-Help

Guided self-help refers to clients using self-help materials with guidance, and there is support for it as a promising, cost-effective, and low-threshold intervention for mild to moderate disordered eating (Traviss-Turner et al., 2017). This guide, though not tailored for guided self-help, can absolutely be used in that way. As discussed in the introduction, one arm of my pilot intervention was guided self-help. Clients received *The Intuitive Eating Workbook* (Tribole & Resch, 2017) and completed one or two chapters of self-study each week. This self-study was supported by a weekly 20-minute phone call with a study "coach," who asked participants about their perceptions of the chapter(s): which content was most helpful and which seemed less applicable. At the end of the calls, the coach assigned the next week's work.

Participants LOVED this modality. They appreciated the flexibility of fitting the self-study into their schedule (rather than attending predetermined sessions), and they really enjoyed processing the content each week with their coach. In fact, we had originally imagined the phone calls would be more of a cursory check-in, but realized participants were really pulling for, and benefiting from, more therapeutic processing. It's amazing what you can accomplish in

20 minutes! In the online resources for this book, I include scripts for conducting guided self-help calls based on *The Intuitive Eating Workbook*. Most of these scripts follow a basic format, but include some notes on potential issues that might arise with each principle.

Telehealth

Telehealth is a growing treatment modality; it increases accessibility and is often more convenient for both clients and providers. Research comparing the effectiveness of treatments delivered via telehealth versus in person is accumulating, and it's promising. Most research suggests comparable or even improved efficacy of treatment delivered virtually versus in person (Shigekawa et al., 2018; Snoswell et al., 2021; Steiger et al., 2022; Torous et al., 2021). I do recommend using technology that enables the use of a whiteboard (or something similar), as visuals can be useful.

With groups, there are advantages and disadvantages to virtual treatment. The convenience means that session attendance will likely increase, but group cohesion and support could suffer due to lack of in-person interaction (this remains untested). I have conducted both in-person and virtual groups and don't perceive one as objectively better than the other: the fit really depends on your group's needs.

Involving Significant Others

Involving supportive significant others in treatment can boost treatment effects. Doing so will depend on the availability and willingness of such people in your client's support system. The acceptance model has shown that unconditional acceptance by others helps people eat more intuitively (Andrew et al., 2014; Augustus-Horvath & Tylka, 2011); it will also be helpful for your client to find people who can model the attitudes and behaviors they are working to adopt. It can be particularly helpful for clients to get support from close others with their between-session exercises and goals each week. For instance, they may want to designate a friend who's willing to eat a feared food with them, or who is someone they can call when they're feeling the urge to engage in a disordered behavior.

If your client's support system is deeply entrenched in diet culture, this support will be harder to come by. It's also possible the people in your client's life will be simply unwilling or unable to support them in working toward a new relationship with eating and body image. If the people in your client's life are more harmful than helpful, work with your client to safely set boundaries and navigate triggering comments and situations. You might also brainstorm how to cultivate a supportive, accepting community outside their immediate circle (e.g., in social media).

Getting Started

As with all clinical practice, you will need to do a thorough intake with your client before getting started. If you're conducting a group, all members should complete the assessment battery before the intervention begins

Intake

If you regularly treat body image and eating-related concerns, your preexisting intake process, including a clinical interview, will likely suffice. Here are factors to assess before initiating intuitive eating treatment specifically:

- Dietary restrictions for medical, religious, ethical, other purposes not related to weight (e.g., low sodium diet, gluten-free, kosher, veganism)

- History of past treatment engagement, including presenting concern, approximate dates, duration, frequency, modality (if known), and perception of benefit

- Comprehensive assessment of current symptoms, including:
  - Trauma history
  - Mood symptoms
  - Suicidal ideation

- Sociodemographic characteristics (including race, ethnicity, immigration status, gender identity, sexual orientation, religion)

- Social support (including living situation and number and quality of current close relationships)

- Employment status (including current work schedule)

- Education status

- Family status (including family composition, number of dependents, caretaking responsibilities)

- Socioeconomic status (including income, healthcare access, insurance coverage, food security)

Assessments

The intake should elucidate your client's primary concerns and treatment goals, which will guide the assessments you choose. I suggest gathering ongoing data to help evaluate progress. At minimum, I recommend assessing your client's level of intuitive eating before and after the intervention. As discussed in Chapter 1, the Intuitive Eating Scale-2 (IES-2) is the most-widely used and empirically validated intuitive eating measure (Tylka & Kroon Van Diest, 2013), and recently had an update (the IES-3; Tylka et al., 2023). Due to the scale's length, it's best used as a comprehensive measure of progress before, midway through, and post intervention). Because we currently lack an empirically validated *brief* intuitive eating measure, you may want to administer a few key items or one of the IES-3 subscales each week. Just note these data would be clinical process data, not necessarily evidence of intervention efficacy.

Whenever possible, choose baseline and outcome measures that are validated for your clients. Because white women have represented the majority of participants in research on body image and eating concerns for decades, many measures were not developed with other groups in mind. For instance, the Eating Disorder Examination (interview and self-report) is one of the most widely used eating-disorder symptom measures (Fairburn & Beglin, 2008), but numerous concerns have been raised about its psychometric validity (Serier, Smith & Yeater, 2018; Goel et al., 2022).

Session Structure

Most of the ten session chapters in this book cover one intuitive eating principle. Because fullness and satisfaction are so interrelated, those principles are covered together in one session, Session 5 (Chapter 8). The last session is spent celebrating progress and future-planning. Sessions follow the original order of the intuitive eating principles, which are designed to build on one another; you may choose to change the order based on your clients' needs.

Each chapter begins with an outline of the content (including materials), an overview of the principle, and the session aim. Some sessions contain additional information about what to expect, either because the principle tends to be a bit challenging or is more likely to elicit defensiveness or difficult group dynamics. Considerations for delivering the content within a group setting are provided. The end of the chapter contains suggestions for how to cover the content across multiple sessions or condense it (e.g., collapsing two principles into one session).

Here is the outline of a typical session.

1. Between-session exercise debriefing (starting in Session 2)
2. Overview of the session's principle
3. Didactic content interspersed with two or three interactive activities
4. Review of upcoming between-session exercises (one to three per week)
5. Session closing

Here's what the typical session components entail and why they are important.

1. Between-Session Exercise Debriefing

All but the first session begin with a quick debriefing on the between-session exercises assigned in the previous session. Debriefing is a great opportunity to hear about and troubleshoot challenges your client or group members encountered, provide feedback, *and* celebrate their wins! Checking in on the exercises also provides some gentle motivation for your client to prioritize them during the week. If your client[13] didn't complete the exercise, troubleshoot what came up. Maybe the exercise didn't resonate with them. Alternatively, the exercise may have generated

---

13 I'll often use the term "client" as a shorthand. If you are leading a group, you can substitute "group members."

fear or discomfort, or the goal turned out to not be feasible or realistic (e.g., planning to track hunger every day, when two or three days would be more feasible).

Ask your client how the exercises went. Did they have any trouble completing them? How helpful were they? Did any exercises *not* resonate? I recommend debriefing each exercise separately so that you can provide feedback and support. If your client feels they didn't do the exercise well "enough," it's important to remind them that the goal is *not* perfection.

In a group setting, give all members an opportunity to share. In a virtual setting, I find "popcorn style," where each group member calls on another member at random to share next, works best. When you leave it open, people are often hesitant to speak up. Though I always emphasize that sharing is voluntary, I also discuss how helpful sharing can be for everyone because it helps to normalize and validate everyone's experiences and brings the group closer. You may structure this part of the session so that group members can provide each other feedback and support. The first sessions may feel a bit awkward as the group warms up to each other, though, in my experience, talking about such personal topics creates a sense of closeness quickly.

2. Introduce the Session's Intuitive Eating Principle(s)

After the debrief, you'll move into introducing the principle you're covering. If the session covers multiple principles, you'll discuss them separately. Introducing the principles is a delicate balance of providing enough information for accurate comprehension without being *too* didactic. Often, this section will involve some reflection and discussion.

3. Present the Week's Content and Interactive Activities

Each topic is accompanied by exercises and/or reflection questions to generate insight and reinforce learning. For instance, when discussing body respect, you'll cover topics like responding to negative body-related comments and self-weighing.

Although you can simply talk through most of the activities, many clients benefit from a visual element. For instance, in Session 1, you and your client can make a list of the ways dieting has negatively interfered with their life. There is something powerful about seeing it written out. For virtual interventions, make use of the whiteboard feature of your conferencing platform or use an online whiteboard. It's often beneficial for your client to take the visual with them: either taking the paper you used or taking a picture of it, or taking a screenshot if you're working online. If you're conducting the intervention in person, I recommend having paper or a whiteboard.

4. Review of Assigned Between-Session Exercises

Before ending the session, you and your client will review the exercises your client will complete before the next session. This is a nice opportunity to make sure you're on the same page.

Determining how many exercises, and which ones to focus on each week should be guided by your clinical judgment and collaboration with your client.

Let clients know, or remind them, that the exercises are designed to put the concepts into action and provide opportunities for practice. Remind them that practice is crucial, as are missteps. Without making mistakes, we're less likely to learn or change. Any profession, hobby, and sport requires considerable time spent *doing*, and that when we practice, we figure out what works, what doesn't, and what can go wrong.

As the intervention progresses, pay attention to the number of exercises that seem to work best for your client. Too few or too infrequent exercises won't optimize their skill-building during the intervention. But *too many* exercises can be overwhelming and probably will not be feasible. What constitutes "not enough" and "too much" depends on the client and can vary week to week. Try to set realistic goals each week, choosing the exercises that are most relevant to your client's concerns. You can always provide more exercises for your client to practice on their own, or you can introduce certain exercises later in the intervention. I like to set SMART goals with my client—that is, goals that are specific, measurable, achievable, realistic, and time-bound. When making a plan for completing the between-session exercises, it's useful to consider what could get in the way and what supports your client may need. For instance, did your client plan to go to an exercise class on a morning after a night out? Perhaps there's another time they could attend the class when they'll be more rested. In terms of social support, would it be helpful for a loved one to know about their goals? If they're doing an activity that might generate fear (e.g., eating a previously off-limits food), would it help to have someone do the exercise with them? Generally, the more concrete and realistic a plan is and the more support and accountability your client has, the more likely they are to meet their goal.

5. Session Closing

I recommend closing each session by asking your client(s) what "hit home" or worked for them from the session. This could be a topic that resonated, a funny or touching moment, or an insight will stick with them. I also recommend that *you* share what hit home for you; in fact, you may want or need to go first to model this reflective practice, especially in the beginning. The closing exercise encapsulates learning and growth and can help your client carry the session with them through the week. In a group setting, this exercise also facilitates group cohesion.

There's no right or wrong way to do this practice, but it might sound something like one of these examples:

- "It hit home for me when Taylor said they laugh less since they started dieting. It really shows how dieting can steal joy."

- "It was powerful to realize how far I've come with body respect. I used to avoid being in pictures. I had to take so many to get even one I didn't hate. Now I jump into pictures with my friends and barely notice my body."

6. Ways to Expand or Condense Session Content

Later in this chapter I provide a general overview of how an intervention may be shortened or lengthened; additionally each session chapter ends with a comprehensive overview of considerations for lengthening or shortening that session.

Each week has several exercises you can do with your clients and several handouts you can provide. Because some exercises and handouts are optional, and treatment length may vary, it can become challenging to keep track of what you did each week and what the client's goals were. A **Session Tracking Log** where you can track each week's exercises, handouts, homework, and goals is included in this manual's online resources. I provide this in two formats: one with a ten-session blueprint, where you can check off the potential exercises, and another that allows you to fill in the details for each session, which may be helpful if you're doing fewer or more than ten sessions.

Shortening Treatment

If treatment must be shortened from ten sessions, suggestions follow for covering the content in four, six, and eight sessions. Fewer than eight sessions have not been empirically evaluated for efficacy. However, shortening treatment may be necessary for a variety of reasons. These guidelines are only suggestions. Some principles may be harder to grasp or more challenging for your client; modify as needed.

Four Sessions

Four sessions is tricky! You'll only have time to briefly introduce each principle, and the sessions will likely be more didactic than interactive. Follow the outline below, or modify it to focus on the principles most relevant to your client's concerns. For instance, if your client struggles with eating in response to emotions and with identifying hunger/fullness cues, but has a healthy relationship with movement and doesn't diet, you may choose to briefly introduce anti-diet principles and skip the content on movement.

Session 1: Ditching Dieting, Honoring Your Hunger, and Fullness and Satisfaction

This is a packed session. You can talk about hunger and fullness together, mentioning satisfaction as a key component of comfortable fullness.

Session 2: Finding Peace with Food and Challenging Thought Patterns

If your client has few food rules or negative food-related cognitions, you may want to move one of the principles from Session 1 here.

Session 3: The Role of Emotions and Body Respect

Session 4: Joyful Movement and Gentle Nutrition

Six Sessions

Session 1: Ditching Dieting and Honoring Hunger

Session 2: Making Peace with Food and Challenging the Food Police

Session 3: Fullness and Satisfaction

Session 4: Coping with Emotions and Body Respect

Session 5: Finding Joy in Movement and Gentle Nutrition

Session 6: Celebrating Progress and Planning for the Future

Eight Sessions

Session 1: Ditching Dieting

Session 2: Honoring Your Hunger

Session 3: Finding Peace with Food and Challenging Thought Patterns

Session 4: Fullness and Satisfaction

Session 5: The Role of Emotions

Session 6: Body Respect

Session 7: Finding Joy in Movement and Gentle Nutrition

Session 8: Celebrating Progress and Planning for the Future

Lengthening Treatment

Becoming an intuitive eater takes time: when it's both indicated and possible, extending treatment is valuable. Here are some factors, specific to each principle, that may merit additional time.

1. Ditching Dieting
   - Lengthy dieting history
   - Doubt or hesitation about intuitive eating
   - Symptoms of orthorexia

Putting the Treatment into Practice

2. Honoring Your Hunger
   - Diminished interoceptive awareness
   - Eating disorder history
   - History of food insecurity
   - Client is an athlete

3. Finding Peace with Food
   - Restrictive eating history or strong cognitive restraint
   - Rigid beliefs about "good" or "bad" foods
   - Client experiences disproportionate weight stigma

4. Challenging Thought Patterns
   - Rigid beliefs about "good" or "bad" foods
   - People in client's support system or family/school/work environment are engaged in dieting or have strong weight-centric beliefs

5. Fullness and Satisfaction
   - History of food insecurity
   - Diminished interoceptive awareness
   - Eating disorder history

6. The Role of Emotions
   - Eating disorder history
   - Co-occurring mental health issues
   - Trauma history

7. Body Respect
   - Most people benefit from extended time with this principle
   - High internalized weight-bias
   - Client experiences disproportionate weight stigma
   - Client participates in an appearance-focused profession or sport
   - Client experiences body dysmorphia

8. Finding Joy in Movement
   - History of disordered exercise
   - Client is or was an athlete
   - Client has a physical disability

9. Gentle Nutrition
   - Most people benefit from extended time with this principle
   - Diminished interoceptive awareness
   - Limited financial resources or food availability

Considerations for Changing the Session Order

The ten intuitive eating principles are designed to build on one another. However, the order is not rigid, and you may change the session order to fit the needs of your client. For instance, if you learn during intake that your client has some degree of body dysmorphia, you might move the session on body respect earlier. Or, while following the sessions in order, you realize something is getting in the way of your client making progress. For instance, you realize in the first session that your client has deeply entrenched beliefs about "good" and "bad" foods, and you decide to work on challenging their rigid food-related beliefs (normally Session 4) before trying to reintroduce feared foods (normally Session 3). Or, your client is making strong progress toward increasing awareness of their hunger cues, and you want to capitalize on this progress by moving immediately to fullness (normally Session 5) before getting into making peace with food and challenging the food police (normally Sessions 3 and 4).

The only principle I suggest you save until later is gentle nutrition (Session 9). If a client is deeply entrenched in diet culture or has rigid beliefs about good or bad foods, it will be quite challenging for them to disentangle whether their motivations for eating nutritious foods are due to how these foods make them feel physically *or* are coming from diet culture. For instance, I've had clients who've done intermittent fasting and keto (without medical necessity) in the past. When they were still making peace with food, we prioritized eating regular meals and snacks that contained adequate carbohydrates. These clients were quick to attribute any feelings of fatigue or brain fog to carbs, likely due to diet culture messaging that carbs make us feel sluggish. These clients were also working mothers of young children: there were *many* potential reasons they experienced fatigue and trouble concentrating. It's possible (even likely) that their food choices sometimes contributed to their not feeling well physically; yet, if making this connection elicited feelings of shame, they likely could work more on their food-related beliefs before focusing on nutrition. So, if your client has a lingering diet mentality or deeply entrenched food beliefs, I advise addressing those before introducing gentle nutrition. Also, that session chapter has an activity to help you and your client determine if they're ready to incorporate gentle nutrition.

You're Ready!

Now that you've learned all about intuitive eating and the nitty-gritty details of the intervention, you're ready to get started! Each of the next ten chapters represents one session and contains all the content and activities you'll need to deliver the intervention. Let's go!

CHAPTER 4

Session 1: Ditching Dieting

Session Outline

Step 1: Introduce Intuitive Eating and Provide a Road Map

Step 2: Encourage Openness and Curiosity

Step 3: Talk a Bit About Weight

　The Open Weight Debate

　Exercise: What If I Didn't Weigh Myself?

Step 4: Define "Diets"

Step 5: Identify the Problem with Diets

　Optional Exercise: Dieting Dissonance

Step 6: Nurture Self-Compassion

　Exercise: Reframing with Self-Compassionate Thoughts

Step 7: Consider the Costs of Micromanaging Eating

　Exercise: How Has Micromanaging My Eating Affected My Life?

　When a Client Is Reluctant to Let Go of Dieting

　Optional Exercise: How Does Dieting Fit with My Values?

Step 8: Between-Session Exercises and Closing

　How Has Micromanaging My Eating Affected My Life?

　Reframing Thoughts with Self-Compassion

　Letting Go of the Tools of Dieting

Materials

Reframing Thoughts with Self-Compassion

How Has Micromanaging My Eating Affected My Life?

Letting Go of the Tools of Dieting

Session Aim

The path toward intuitive eating starts with dislodging what we've learned about food and bodies ("diet culture"[14]) from its entrenched place in many of our brains, which are formed in Westernized and colonized cultures. Thus, the intuitive eating principle Reject Diet Culture is, crucially, the first.

When we spend our lives absorbing countless messages about which bodies are acceptable and how we need to eat and move to achieve said bodies, we're unlikely to question these messages or look beyond them unless we're given a reason to do so. Before clients can begin to make peace with food and honor their body cues, they must first become aware of, and then start to reject, diet culture messages.

What Are Diets?

In intuitive eating work, "diets" mean ANY set of non-medically necessary rules about how much, when, or what to eat. Sometimes diets are marketed as such (e.g., the Atkins diet). In recent years, diets often masquerade as "lifestyle" or "wellness" programs. These are still diets, and they're not compatible with intuitive eating. Many diets involve cutting out specific foods or entire food groups (e.g., low/no sugar, low/no carb). Some recommend restricting eating to certain times of day, or even alternating days of eating with days of fasting. What these diets all have in common is the presumption that individuals cannot or should not trust the innate wisdom of their bodies, and that rigid rules are needed to achieve health, happiness, or beauty. Vegetarianism, veganism, gluten-free, and religious dietary rules (such as halal or kosher), among others, are in a separate category, and can be compatible with intuitive eating. However, sometimes these diets *can* conceal a budding or fully developed eating disorder. A thorough assessment, differentiating ethical or medically indicated diets from rule-based diets in disguise, is a crucial pre-intervention step, particularly in the context of individual therapy (see Chapter 3).

Throughout the manual, I use "dieting" as shorthand. If this term does't work for your client or group members, use whatever terminology will resonate with them. (One I have found salient for college women is "micromanaging your eating.")

What to Expect from This Session

Chances are, clients in middle to late adulthood will immediately recognize and understand the term "diet." However, "diet" often feels dated for younger generations, evoking images of SlimFast shakes and Jenny Craig. With younger people, you may need to spend more time unpacking what diets are and what they look like now. And even people born before 2000, who will likely be

---

[14] I refer to "diet culture" given its familiarity to most who work in the intuitive eating space. However, it's a term that oversimplifies the racist origins of anti-fat bias, so when I use it, please read it with that perspective in mind.

familiar with the term, may be unaware of the insidious ways diets show up in culture today. I've included an optional exercise, Dieting Dissonance, to help clients gain awareness of diet trends.

Reactions to this session can vary depending on a client's background and history. I've seen every reaction from clear and immediate relief to defensiveness and skepticism. For those with long histories of dieting and repeated attempts at weight loss, this principle may feel like freedom. For clients who've been told by medical professionals that they *need* to lose weight for their health, it can evoke fear and skepticism. I have also observed doubt and hesitation among women fixated on "healthy" eating who had symptoms reflective of orthorexia.

As discussed in Chapter 3, the theory of psychological reactance posits that when people feel their freedom or choices are threatened, they may act in opposition to regain a sense of control. So, it's crucial in this first session to encourage openness and avoid a heavy hand. Intuitive eating is about self-care, flexibility, and honoring one's needs. There's no one right way to be an intuitive eater. Throughout these sessions, encourage your clients to learn what helps them meet their unique physical and emotional needs.

Additional Considerations and Potential Adaptations

Many people diet to make their bodies feel safer to inhabit—the desire for weight loss or fear of weight gain is often not about simple body dissatisfaction. For instance, some Black women may feel safer existing in a body that aligns with white, Eurocentric standards of respectability, beauty, and status. In such circumstances, dieting is less about body dissatisfaction than about *survival*.

Body image concerns are often driven by the same structural and social factors that place Black, Brown, trans, nonbinary, female, disabled, and fat bodies at increased risk of violence. This doesn't mean we can't help our clients move toward body respect, but it *does* mean we need to be aware of what letting go of dieting may represent to our clients, particularly when we encounter fear or resistance. Encountering fear or resistance can help us and our client discern what ditching dieting represents to the client.

For clients with eating disorder histories, this principle may feel less salient. Eating disorders may start with a well-intentioned or even recommended attempt at dieting or weight loss. However, the etiology of eating disorders is biopsychosocial, extending far beyond the pursuit of weight loss and/or appearance ideals. Use your clinical judgment to guide how much time to spend unpacking and exploring the harms of dieting. Instead, you may choose to shift your focus to discussing how eating disorder thoughts, attitudes, and/or behaviors have impacted their life. This exploration should be done with the utmost compassion. Your client didn't choose to have an eating disorder. However, if they're seeking treatment, it's likely they realize the eating disorder is no longer working for them. This first session is the perfect time to begin that exploration. As mentioned in Chapter 3, having clinical expertise in eating disorder treatment or supervision by someone with such expertise is crucial if you're working with a client with an active eating disorder or one in recovery.

> ### Considerations for Group Interventions
>
> As you'll see, there's a lot to introduce in this first session. For many clients, intuitive eating concepts will be totally new, or may have reached your clients in distorted form. Thus, in a group there is a greater risk of members saying things that are potentially triggering to other members, are inaccurate, or are contradictory to intuitive eating. Knowing this, you may be tempted to make the first session more didactic to prevent group members from latching onto messages that run counter to intuitive eating. Yet, the first session is also when participants are most likely to be shy and hesitant, and when the risk of drop-out is highest. So I recommend that you balance informative content with enough interaction to allow group members to begin developing a sense of cohesion. I recommend telling the group in the first session that the leaders will highlight (with compassion) any comments made that are misaligned with intuitive eating, and that this is done to deepen learning within the group.

Step 1: Introduce Intuitive Eating and Provide a Road Map

After introductions, begin orienting your client to intuitive eating. They likely have some notion of what intuitive eating entails if they agreed to engage with it, so your overview needn't be expansive. However, it's helpful to briefly survey intuitive eating's core components and provide a roadmap of where the client is headed.

Before you introduce the principles, I recommend highlighting that intuitive eating is a framework that covers eating, body image, and movement. I like to convey that intuitive eating's principles touch on:

- rethinking dieting
- getting in touch with your body's needs
- letting go of food-related rules and beliefs that are no longer working for you
- fostering adaptive coping skills
- learning to distinguish between physical and emotional needs
- developing a more peaceful body image
- finding forms of movement that feel good
- reexamining nutrition in your food choices

You might give some background about the origins of intuitive eating and how it has gained momentum and research support over time.

Let clients know the principles are arranged in order because they build on and support each other, so you'll be covering one or two principles each week (however many your intervention is structured for—see Chapter 3). Tell them this structure is designed to give them time to learn to apply each principle before moving on to the next. Again, this part of the session can be brief, but it helps to orient clients to what's ahead.

Step 2: Encourage Openness and Curiosity

Openness and curiosity are important attitudes to encourage and model throughout the intervention. The risk of skepticism, defensiveness, and fear is highest in the first sessions, and it's essential that clients feel their rights of autonomy and agency are respected. This is in keeping with the spirit of intuitive eating—of gaining awareness of and beginning to trust one's own needs. Modeling an open, curious approach while encouraging your clients to be open and curious as they consider what feels "right" for *them* is a beautiful opportunity for attunement.

So, right after introducing intuitive eating, explicitly encourage your client to greet any information they learn throughout the intervention with openness and curiosity. Acknowledge and affirm that not all the content will feel personally applicable, and some may generate feelings of skepticism. Encourage them to explore any emotional reactions they have, now and throughout the intervention. Ask them to wonder what might be underneath the feelings coming up. When your client's autonomy is honored from the very beginning, and they don't experience pressure to change their beliefs, they'll feel safer exploring them.

For you, this is a delicate balance to maintain throughout the intervention. Some attitudes and beliefs simply aren't aligned with intuitive eating; others may be downright harmful. Perhaps a client who struggles to stop eating when full mentions they have started to brush their teeth to prevent eating more (an idea that likely came from diet culture "wisdom"). As this could easily become a disordered behavior, your clinical judgment might suggest being more direct with this client, perhaps providing some psychoeducation or asking open-ended, curious questions, and offering alternate ideas to navigate urges to eat when full.

Step 3: Talk a Bit About Weight

Weight should be acknowledged at the beginning of the intervention.[15] Most clients will have complicated, often difficult thoughts and feelings about weight. Some may be holding out hope that embarking upon intuitive eating will lead to weight loss. Others may be hoping they won't *gain* weight. Regardless of the client's history with and feelings about weight, this is the moment to provide education about why weight *won't* be the focus at any point during the intervention.

---

15 As a reminder, individuals in active weight restoration may be introduced to intuitive eating but should be scaffolded carefully (see Chapter 2). Those in eating disorder recovery will need additional support and time to reestablish connection and trust with their bodies and bodily cues. Intuitive eating is appropriate for those firmly rooted in recovery, medically stable, and weight restored. Target weights should be individualized and based on a person's individual growth trajectory. For more, see Steinberg et al. (2023).

You want to begin the work of helping clients become aware of and disentangle from what may be deeply rooted beliefs, including the idea that weight directly reflects one's health and behaviors. Further, you want to touch on how self-weighing could derail the work your client is doing to heal their relationship with food and body image. Guided by your clinical judgment, begin to explore with clients the ways that weight is complex, with biological, genetic, social, environmental, and behavioral origins (Bacon et al., 2011; Rubino et al., 2020). Some topics to touch on may include the following.

1. Weight is complex, but it's often simplified into a (frequently inaccurate) measure of health status, or seen as a result of eating and exercise behaviors. These ideas aren't helpful; in fact, they hurt people.

2. Attributions of personal responsibility and the controllability of weight help drive weight bias (Black et al., 2014; Brownell et al., 2010). When weight is seen as controllable and as each person's individual responsibility, and when higher weight is conflated with poor health, high-weight people are subject to judgment and shame.

3. If weight were truly controllable, surely the billions of dollars spent on weight management interventions over the last decades would have yielded marked and *sustained* weight loss among participants. Yet, an infinitesimal minority of people maintain significant weight loss over the *long term* (Nordmo et al., 2020).

4. BMI is an inherently flawed tool, oversimplified and misused. Consider recommending *Fearing the Black Body* by Sabrina Strings to clients; it includes a history of the racist origins of anti-fat bias and the body mass index (BMI). BMI is not the direct reflection of health we're told it is. Some people at higher BMIs engage in health-promoting behaviors and are metabolically healthy, just as some people at lower BMIs do not and are not. Although weight can sometimes provide *some* information about

The Open Weight Debate

There is controversy in the eating disorder field around *open weighing*: regularly weighing clients and allowing them to see the number. Proponents argue that this is essential exposure that helps break the fear/avoidance cycle. Others, acknowledging how laden with meaning weight has become in our culture, are more cautious. For some clients, especially those in larger bodies, repeatedly being exposed to a number that is labeled as wrong or diseased can be traumatic.

I tend to side with the cautious approach. As noted in Chapter 3, this program is not appropriate for someone in early recovery from an eating disorder. Even so, diet- and weight-related beliefs are likely deeply entrenched for most other clients, and dislodging those beliefs takes time and practice. If, early in this program, a client steps on the scale and sees an upward trend, they may become skeptical of intuitive eating and want to retreat to behaviors that offer the allure of weight maintenance or loss. I've witnessed this phenomenon in my clinical work. For that reason, I discourage self-weighing with my clients unless it's medically necessary.

health status (e.g., sudden weight change due to a medical condition), it's a small piece of a much bigger picture and should be understood as such.

Your clients may be skeptical, and that's OK! You're encouraging them to reflect on alternate perspectives to figure out what feels right to them. You may also have clients who are concerned their weight status will lead to negative health effects now or in the future. I like to redirect clients to focusing on what we *do* have some influence over, including behaviors. Weight is not a behavior, nor a dial that can be turned up or down. Health improvements can occur in the absence of weight changes. For instance, working with a PT or beginning some gentle yoga or mobility work could help clients dealing with joint pain. For clients with prediabetes, dietary changes can be made in the context of intuitive eating. Taking the focus off weight just makes sense given we don't directly control it and it doesn't tell the whole story.

It's crucial when working with clients in larger bodies that *you* recognize the disproportionate stigma and challenges they face, especially if they're carrying other marginalized identities. Don't reassure your clients that they won't gain weight, as this reinforces the idea that gaining weight is a negative outcome, when it's a neutral outcome in intuitive eating. Similarly, don't suggest that clients may *lose* weight. It's simply not possible to know how someone's body will respond to intuitive eating. Your job is to help clients build a new relationship with their bodies, one characterized by trust in their bodies and an appreciation for what their bodies do, not based on their bodies' size or appearance.

Finally, I discourage using the terms "overweight" or "obese" as they can cause distress and harm. See Meadows and Daníelsdóttir (2016) for more on the problems with these terms. If your client is fat, ask them about their preferred terms!

EXERCISE: What If I Didn't Weigh Myself?

If your client engages in self-weighing, consider exploring how this behavior could affect their progress toward intuitive eating. Self-weighing can derail intuitive eating by tempting clients to change their eating habits in reaction to the number. For instance, if your client steps on the scale and sees a lower number than expected, they may feel relief (if desiring weight loss) or anger (if desiring weight or muscle gain). They may feel tempted to modify their behaviors to maintain, increase, or reduce the number. Similarly, seeing a higher number on the scale may generate feelings of fear, shame, or relief. These emotions can motivate restriction or bulking behaviors. It's easy to see how the message given by the number on the scale is rarely neutral: it's not information your client can rely on to guide their eating, as it's unrelated to their body's needs. The goal of this exercise is to help clients see that self-weighing will likely slow or halt their intuitive eating progress. We'll revisit this exercise in Session 7 (Body Respect), so if you perceive that your client's self-weighing practices won't interfere with their intuitive eating work, you can save this until then.

For clients who don't regularly weigh themselves but also haven't committed to *not* doing so, you may still reflect on how self-weighing can disrupt intuitive eating. If your client has already done the work to reduce or stop self-weighing, you can skip this. Some clients may feel neutral toward their weight already, in that seeing the number *doesn't* affect how they eat. In this case: excellent! This exercise may be less relevant.

Some clients *must* weigh themselves for medical reasons (e.g., to monitor fluid balance). If these clients have complicated feelings about their weight, you can help them process that. And it may be helpful if a loved one can assist these clients with weighing if the number feels charged for them. Skipping weighing shouldn't be a goal for these clients.

If you're short on time, skip the more extensive questions below and explore what it would be like for clients to consider not weighing themselves for a week.

> Think of the last time you stepped on the scale. What feelings came up *before* you stepped on?
>
> Once you saw the number, how did you feel?
>
> How did seeing your weight affect how you ate?
>> If the number was higher than you expected or hoped, imagine stepping on the scale and seeing a *lower* number than expected. How might it affect how you ate?
>>
>> If the number was lower than you expected or hoped, imagine stepping on the scale and seeing a *higher* number than expected. How might it affect how you ate?
>
> What would it be like to stop weighing yourself? What feelings come up when you think about stopping?
>
> Imagine what it might be like if you were free to meet your body's needs without needing to micromanage your behaviors for the sake of your shape or size. What is it like when the number on the scale no longer dictates how you get to eat and move?

I like to wrap up this activity by setting a goal with the client. You might encourage clients who weigh themselves to take a week off, with a plan to notice what the experience is like for them. If that feels like too much, you can start slower (check out the **Graduated Exposure** exercise in Session 3 for ideas on how to build toward a bigger, scary goal). Some clients may not be ready to ditch the scale yet. Being overbearing on this point could create reactivity, so it's OK to plant seeds and revisit the topic later.

Step 4: Define "Diets"

Here, you get clients on the same page regarding the word "diet." Start by exploring what a diet is to them. What does the word bring to mind? What are their general attitudes toward dieting? Even if your clients seem quite familiar with diets, it's still useful to establish a working definition that you'll use for the remainder of your work together. If the word "diet" doesn't resonate with your client, use a term that does, such as "lifestyle change" or "routine."

A diet involves any non-medically necessary rules about how much, when, and/or what to eat. As noted, religious practices such as keeping kosher or observing Ramadan are not diets, nor are choices made for ethical reasons, such as not eating meat. However, it's important to explore

Session 1: Ditching Dieting

your client's history and relationship with these practices, as they can mask disordered eating patterns.

If you ask your client what they think of when they hear the word "diet" and the only examples they generate are from the distant past (e.g., Jenny Craig), it'll be important to spend a little more time discussing current dieting trends. If you think your client understands what a "diet" is in the context of intuitive eating, you can move on to the next topic.

Step 5: Identify the Problem with Diets

Once clients have a working definition of diets, it's time to walk through why intuitive eating is an anti-diet framework. Ultimately, the human body is not made for diets. We're biologically primed to stay nourished, and our bodies almost always fight against dieting. When food is scarce, the body works to conserve resources and find nourishment (Galgani & Santos, 2016; MacLean et al., 2004). Because the body doesn't know when adequate food will be available again, metabolism slows, and biological processes not essential for survival (e.g., menstruation) may be suspended. You're more likely to notice food-related cues in your environment and to find food more rewarding (Demos et al., 2011; Stice et al., 2013). These mechanisms are adaptive, helping you survive.

Many diets, like paleo and intermittent fasting, are marketed as "getting back to our ancestral roots." Proponents argue that we evolved to fast because our ancestors were forced to endure periods of famine. They omit that it's unnatural to deprive ourselves of food if we're hungry and it's available. It's unlikely that, outside of religious or spiritual contexts, our ancestors were depriving themselves of available food when they experienced the desire to eat.

Tailor this content to your client, with a goal of helping them realize that they haven't failed diets, diets have failed *them*. Although dieting, disordered eating, and eating disorders share many symptoms and attitudes, they're *not* the same, so this conversation will look different depending on the person and their history. With someone who has frequently dieted with the goal of weight loss, you may want to highlight that very few people (3 to 5 percent) achieve sustained weight loss long-term, and even when they do, it may come at a psychological or physical cost (Spirou, Raman & Smith, 2020; Nordmo, Danielsen & Nordmo, 2020). And dramatic weight loss can have lingering negative consequences. For instance, research on the long-term outcomes of the Biggest Loser

> We *never* want to use the link between dieting and weight gain to fearmonger. It's perfectly fine to acknowledge that diets very rarely achieve the intended goal of long-term: we make this point mainly to emphasize the futility of dieting. However, the reason we want clients to stop dieting is *not* so they avoid weight gain, but to help them leave a distressing, harmful cycle that doesn't serve their long-term health and limits their power to live full, authentic lives.

contestants found that, even six years later, contestants' metabolisms and leptin levels (the "fullness" hormone) remained suppressed and lost muscle was not regained (Fothergill et al., 2016).

You may have clients who have participated in eating trends or dieting fads with other motivations, such as health or wellness. Wellness trends are often driven by pseudoscience and rely on shaky, misconstrued, or overgeneralized data. It's common to see, for example, a news article extolling the benefits of intermittent fasting, citing one research study that was conducted on three white men over nine months. Sigh.

Some questions you might ask your client during this conversation:

1. How often in the past did you feel you failed when you didn't stick to a diet?
2. What would it be like to consider that maybe the diets failed you?

OPTIONAL EXERCISE: Dieting Dissonance

In this dissonance-based exercise, you ask your client to argue *against* dieting. In an individual session, you might role-play the part of a friend who is thinking about starting a new diet. Your client's job is to ask clarifying questions and help you see why a diet is likely not the best idea. This exercise works well in a group. Depending on group size, you can either have members pair off *or* you and your co-facilitator can take turns playing the friend who wants to diet. Group members can then each try to persuade you, or their conversation partner, to not diet.

The goal of this exercise is not to bash diets, but to practice expressing the reasons why dieting is likely to be futile or even ultimately harmful. If you don't have time for this exercise in session, your client can write a letter or email to a friend expressing concerns about their plan to diet.

Step 6: Nurture Self-Compassion

Cultivating self-compassion is an essential part of becoming an intuitive eater. Most folks I've worked with have brutal self-critics in their heads. And research shows a strong link between shame and disordered eating (Nechita et al., 2021). Clients may feel their inner critic helps them achieve their goals; but it's more than likely the critic is keeping them stuck. Instead, as one's self-compassion goes up, one's disordered eating and body image distress go down (Braun et al., 2016). Among other benefits, self-compassion can help protect people when they encounter threats to their body image and eating, like appearance-focused content on social media (Tylka & Kroon Van Diest, 2015).

When we're learning something new, our automatic thoughts are often self-critical. Growth is hard! It's easy to forget that missteps, stumbles, and falls are *necessary* for learning. Eating past fullness, for example, is useful for learning what that sensation feels like—and realizing it's not very comfortable. Similarly, forgetting to carry a snack and getting overly hungry is going to be memorable. Either event could be an occasion for self-blame or shame, but self-compassion lets us see these events as good information that can help us make other choices in the future. Self-critical thoughts can disrupt learning, so help your client learn to reframe them with self-compassion. This is a skill, and it will take practice; remind clients that any time they're learning a new way of doing or being, it's likely to feel unnatural and effortful. Let them know this is OK—then help them practice!

EXERCISE: Reframing with Self-Compassionate Thoughts

This exercise is designed to give clients practice reframing self-critical thoughts into self-compassionate ones. In an individual session, you can simply ask the questions below. In a group, you may have group members pair off and ask each other these questions as a role-play exercise.

1. *Think of a recent critical thought you have had about food, eating, or body image. What did this inner dialogue sound like?*

    People are often harsh with themselves about how they perceive their body and how they eat. These thoughts may be so rehearsed that your client is on autopilot and not even aware of how self-critical their thoughts are. Generating awareness is an important first step to cognitive reframing. An example of an automatic self-critical thought could be, "I can't believe I ate so much. I feel so gross."

2. *Picture that someone in your life you feel particularly close to is in this exact situation. How would it feel to hear them speak to themself this way?*

    Often, it's painful to imagine a loved one speaking to themself the way we speak to ourselves. Although we often think we deserve negative self-talk, we *rarely* think a loved one should be so harsh on themself.

3. *What would you say to your friend in this situation? How might you encourage them to modify their self-talk?*

    While we often display all-or-nothing thinking with ourselves and lose the nuance of a situation, we're usually able to see context and generate empathy for others. For instance, clients might offer to a friend, "It's really uncomfortable to eat past fullness, but you did nothing wrong." Clients might also normalize for their friend that almost everyone eats past fullness sometimes, and reflect how these moments when we feel a little too hungry or too full provide useful information. Maybe next time we remind ourselves to pack a snack, or we try to eat a bit more slowly.

After this exercise, debrief! What was different about how they speak to themselves versus someone they care about? What was it like to practice more self-compassionate thoughts? Clients may reflect that trying to reframe critical thoughts with compassionate ones feels clunky, awkward, or unnatural. Reflect back to them that, after a lifetime of rehearsing self-critical thoughts, it makes sense when self-compassionate ones are not top of mind.

Because self-compassion is not the default for most, it will require practice. For that reason, I recommend taking a moment to return to this exercise during sessions when clients express self-critical thoughts to reinforce learning. It's also a great early goal to practice this exercise between sessions. In the free tools at http://www.newharbinger.com/52540, you'll find a **Reframing Thoughts with Self-Compassion** handout for clients.

Step 7: Consider the Costs of Micromanaging Eating

Your client's growing awareness of the costs of micromanaging their eating (dieting) should create the dissonance that can help motivate change. Often these behaviors and obsessions are on autopilot, and we can't change what we don't see! This exercise is intended to get clients thinking about the ways dieting may be harming their life, be in conflict with their values, or be getting in the way of their goals. Lead them through the questions, each of which is accompanied by considerations you can use to prompt or guide the conversation. If you're running short on time in session, model the first question or two with your client, then give them the take-home version of this exercise.

EXERCISE: How Has Micromanaging My Eating Affected My Life?

1. **How does micromanaging eating impact your social life?**

   Do they turn down social invitations because of food- or body image–related fears? Do they bring their own food, or eat things they don't really want?[16] Do body image concerns affect their romantic relationships? Is their enjoyment of social activities diminished because they struggle with food and body image?

2. **How does micromanaging eating impact your mental and physical health?**

   Does dieting affect their mood, energy, or sleep? Do they notice physical symptoms, such as fatigue or lightheadedness, related to dieting?

3. **How does micromanaging eating impact resources such as time, money, and physical or mental energy?**

   This question gets at some hidden costs of dieting. Clients may not realize how much time, energy, and money they expend on dieting.

4. **What hopes do you have about what will happen if you could control your eating or if you reach a certain shape or size?[17]**

   Clients may believe their lives will improve, or desired things will happen, once they've reached a certain weight, shape, or size, or can control their eating.

5. **What aspects of your life have you put on hold until you reach these goals?**

---

16 Some clients may not feel safe eating certain foods in public. Whereas someone in a thin body can eat ice cream in public with little risk of discrimination, the same cannot be said for someone in a large body.

17 For clients with eating disorder histories, behaviors and attitudes are unlikely to be rooted in fantasies about having a thinner body. Rather, the eating disorder may feel safe, and the future unknown. Here, you may instead explore what the client is afraid of giving up. What fears come up when imagining a future without the eating disorder? Similarly, if your client's dieting is rooted in oppression and the desire for safety, this question could appear to minimize that reality. You may want to stay focused on whether the costs outweigh the potential benefits.

Clients may not realize they're perpetually putting their lives on hold for reasons related to body image and dieting goals. They may not be dating because they feel unworthy, or are worried potential partners won't find them attractive. Others may avoid intimacy with partners.[18] They may put off buying clothing until they reach a certain size, avoid fashions they think their bodies are not meant for, or avoid activities involving swimsuits.

Many people believe they'll start intuitive eating or work on body respect once they reach a certain body shape or size. However, you cannot truly embrace intuitive eating if you are working to maintain a shape or size your body isn't meant to be. Further, bodies are meant to change throughout the lifespan! Realistically, will a person ever *really* be able to start eating intuitively if they're waiting until they're a certain weight or shape? What happens as their bodies age and change?

This exercise comes with a handout (**How Has Micromanaging My Eating Affected My Life?**) that clients can complete between sessions.

It's critical to acknowledge that part of the reality weight stigma creates is that some aspects of life *do* get easier when one is in a smaller body. People *may* treat you differently, you *may* get more attention from potential romantic partners, and different opportunities *may* exist. If you yourself are in a smaller body, it's your task to stay aware of how weight-related oppression shows up in myriad ways you are likely privileged to not have to notice (clothes shopping, public transportation). Ignorance of issues of weight-related oppression can harm your clients. Some clients will need more support for coping with weight-related oppression; extend treatment if that is accessible. Learning to trust and accept one's body is a radical act in a world that punishes and shames most bodies (especially those that are fat, Black, Brown, trans, and/or disabled). Acknowledging this is critical for clients who experience disproportionate stigma.

When a Client Is Reluctant to Let Go of Dieting

When clients feel particularly reluctant to let dieting go, I ask them to project out far into the future. How do they imagine they'll feel at age eighty, for example, looking back and seeing a life dedicated to micromanaging eating and/or attaining a certain body shape or size? How do they think they'll wish they had spent their valuable time and resources?

---

18 Your client may have a partner who doesn't accept their body. Being in a partnership where one's desirability and acceptability depends on being a certain shape or weight will merit exploration.

OPTIONAL EXERCISE: How Does Dieting Fit with My Values?

Another exercise for reluctant clients involves making a values pie chart. This will be familiar to clinicians with training in CBT-E (enhanced cognitive behavioral therapy). With your client, generate a list of their top values (e.g., family, relationships, work, spending time outdoors). Then, create a pie chart assigning each value to a slice of the pie. Use percentages to denote the relative importance of each value; for instance, perhaps family takes up one-third of the pie, whereas work is just 10 percent. Note these are values the person holds but may not necessarily live into: aspirational values.

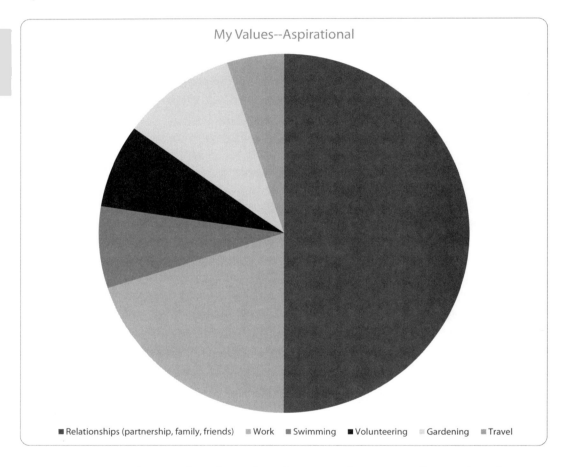

Now create another pie chart that reflects how your client is actually spending their time and resources. Compare this to their aspirational-values pie chart; specifically, what resources are they expending on food and body image, and does this align with their values?

Session 1: Ditching Dieting

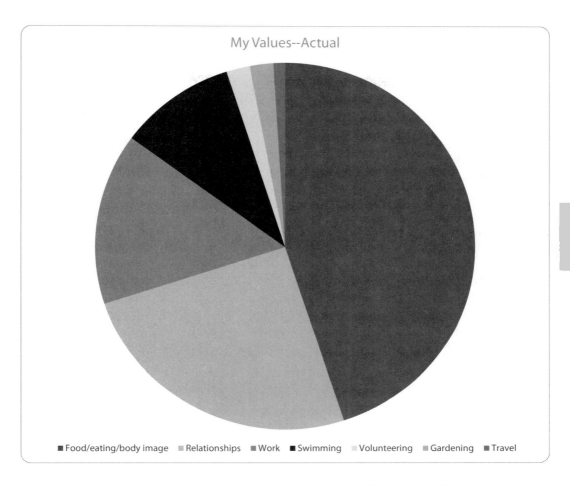

This exercise can be jarring, but the goal is *not* to generate shame. In a culture saturated with messages about how we should eat and look, it makes sense that people may expend considerable resources to micromanage their eating and/or their bodies. Maintain an empathic stance throughout this exercise. The goal is to generate insight and, ideally, just enough dissonance to motivate change. When clients realize they're not living a life aligned with their values, they can then consider what needs to change to bring these back into alignment.

Step 8: Between-Session Exercises and Closing

There are three between-session exercises for this week; choose the one (or more) that you judge will help clients most at this point.

The **How Has Micromanaging My Eating Affected My Life?** handout asks clients to create an inventory of, and then reflect on, the ways dieting has interfered with their lives. The goal of this reflection is to crystallize the concepts discussed in session and generate further dissonance to propel change, *not* to fuel shame. If you feel this exercise would be more distressing than helpful for your client, save it for later or skip it entirely.

The **Reframing Thoughts with Self-Compassion** handout provides clients with more opportunities to practice self-compassion, which likely most clients could use.

Finally, because dieting is deeply embedded in our culture, clients may not recognize how the dieting tools they use in their daily lives might be harmful. Keeping a calorie tracking app on our phones, for instance, could be a powerful cue that draws us back to old, destructive patterns. The **Letting Go of the Tools of Dieting** worksheet lists common dieting tools and tricks, with space for clients to add their own. For homework, clients can choose at least one dieting tool they will practice letting go of between sessions. For some, letting go of the most salient or prominent tool (e.g., following fitness influencers on social media) may be the most therapeutic option (think: flooding). However, some may not be ready or have the support to let go of their most-used tools. You might help those clients identify an intermediate step they can take in letting go, and document their plan on the worksheet.

Closing

Close the session by summarizing the discussion and asking your client what worked for them from the session. This exercise can help clients carry these principles with them through the week and encapsulate learning and growth. If they are hesitant to share, you can go first!

Session 1: Ditching Dieting

Lengthening the Session

If time and resources permit, this session can be expanded into two. This may be especially helpful if your client:

- Has a history of an eating disorder
- Has a lengthy history of dieting or weight cycling
- Grew up around dieting or has loved ones with deeply entrenched beliefs about dieting
- Displays orthorexia behaviors (which they may not see as dieting)
- Is skeptical of intuitive eating

To lengthen into two sessions:

- Spend most of the first session discussing dieting, your client's dieting history, and the reasons why intuitive eating is anti-diet.
- Spend most of the second session on practicing self-compassion and exploring the costs of dieting for clients' lives.

Shortening the Session

If you need to shorten this session, do a briefer introduction to diets, and focus on practicing self-compassion and exploring the costs of dieting (especially as they manifest for your client). Spend less time on how diets show up today and the research behind the problems with dieting. Some of the general problems with dieting will become apparent as clients explore how dieting harms *their own* lives. Your clients' relationship with the scale should guide how much time you spend discussing weight; if clients have a neutral relationship with the scale, you may need less time on the material. However, if clients engage in frequent self-weighing or feel deeply invested in their weight, beginning to unpack that is important.

CHAPTER 5

Session 2: Honoring Your Hunger

Session Outline

Step 1: Between-Session Exercises Debriefing

    How Has Micromanaging My Eating Affected My Life?

    Reframing Thoughts with Self-Compassion

    Letting Go of the Tools of Dieting

Step 2: Explore the What and Why of Hunger

    Exercise: Hunger Is Just Another Cue

Step 3: Body-Cue Awareness

Step 4: How Does Your Hunger Speak to You?

    Exercise: Discovering Hunger

    Handout: Hunger Rating Scale

    Handout: Hunger Discovery Log

Step 5: Distinguishing Hunger Cues from Thoughts and Other Inputs

    Handout: Mind, Body Cue, or Self-Care

Step 6: What Gets in the Way of Hunger?

    Handout: Self-Care Assessment

Step 7: Between-Session Exercises and Closing

    Hunger Discovery Log

    Hunger Rating Scale

    Self-Care Log

Materials

Hunger Rating Scale

Hunger Discovery Log

Mind, Body Cue, or Self-Care

Self-Care Assessment

Self-Care Log

Session 2: Honoring Your Hunger

Session Aim

This session is all about, you guessed it, hunger! Specifically, you'll be helping clients identify potential barriers to detecting their hunger cues, learn how hunger shows up in *their* body, and begin to distinguish thoughts from physiological signals. The overarching aim is that your client moves toward using their hunger cues to help guide their eating. That is, clients will better understand how they experience hunger, know what barriers might get in the way, and use their hunger to help guide what, when, and how much they eat.

Remember: intuitive eating is never all-or-nothing. Sometimes clients will *need* to eat when they're not hungry, and sometimes they will simply choose to. Hunger may present in less obvious ways for some clients (e.g., irritability), or it may continue to feel elusive—both of which can make this principle challenging. Although eating by hunger is what intuitive eating is primarily known for in popular culture, it's just one of ten principles. Your goal is to help your clients cultivate attunement, *if* that is accessible to them, so that eating by hunger is a tool they reach for much of the time.

What to Expect from This Session

In my experience, this principle resonates with many clients (with exceptions detailed below). In particular, the importance of self-care and how it interacts with hunger strikes a chord. It can be incredibly healing to be given permission to prioritize your well-being. However, some people have learned to associate hunger with shame. Being hungry can feel like a sign of weakness or like an annoyance. It's tragic that diet culture and anti-fatness are so powerful they render people fearful of the cues their bodies use to communicate their needs. Normalizing and contextualizing hunger is central to this principle, and this session.

Clients aren't always aware of how hunger shows up in their bodies. Many associate hunger with their stomach growling (what I call "tummy hunger") or with a sensation of emptiness. However, some may experience hunger differently, and may have never connected feeling tired or foggy, for instance, with needing sustenance. It can be challenging to sort out and make sense of all the various internal experiences we have going on! Clients may struggle to differentiate a genuine physiological hunger cue from an emotion or a thought. This issue will be covered toward the end of the session and will be the topic of a between-session exercise.

Additional Considerations and Potential Adaptations

It's likely you'll encounter clients with diminished interoceptive awareness, low appetite, or early satiety. Interoceptive awareness is often altered in the context of eating disorders (and there is debate about whether differences[19] in interoceptive awareness precipitate or are a consequence

---

19   I try to avoid the term "deficits," which implies inadequacy or insufficiency and feels unnecessarily judgment-laden.

of disordered eating). Interoceptive awareness may improve with nutritional rehabilitation and consistent intake. However, as noted in Chapter 2, clients' readiness to begin using their hunger and fullness cues to guide eating varies. Some clients in recovery from disordered eating may wish to retain some structure to their eating to avoid relapse. Interoceptive cues may also be diminished by certain medical conditions and treatments (e.g., chemotherapy). In these cases, an interdisciplinary team (dietitian, therapist, physician) can help ensure the patient's needs are understood and met. Finally, there is evidence that some neurodivergent populations, including autistic people and those with ADHD, have differences in their awareness and integration of interoceptive cues (Hatfield et al., 2019; Kutscheidt et al., 2019) compared to neurotypical people. In any of these cases, collaborate with your client and use your clinical judgment to guide how you approach this principle. In *most* circumstances, I think it's useful to explore interoception with clients. There are various ways our bodies communicate to us; these may not always align with our expectations. However, when it may not make sense for clients to use their hunger cues to determine when or even how much to eat, skip activities or content you judge not pertinent or helpful.

I structured this session so that, first, clients are oriented to why we experience hunger. Then, they begin to focus on how *they* experience hunger and on distinguishing biological hunger from thoughts and self-care needs (we'll address emotions in a later session). At the end, you'll discuss self-care and identify what can get in the way of or facilitate experiencing hunger cues.[20]

Considerations for Group Interventions

When conducting this intervention in a group setting, I have group members go around and discuss their reasons for signing up in the second session. In the first session, there is so much to go over, and nerves tend to be high. It takes a little time for folks to warm up and feel comfortable speaking. However, sharing why they joined the group can be a way to bond and feel seen. The main consideration with this exercise is to keep in mind how power dynamics could show up. For instance, heterogeneous groups can engender social comparison. Clients in smaller bodies or engaging in restrictive behaviors may feel more comfortable sharing their reasons for signing up because of the social capital assigned to thinness and restriction. Balancing these dynamics will be important for group leaders to maintain safety.

If the group seems hesitant to share, facilitators can discuss how their own interest in intuitive eating developed, *provided* that the self-disclosure is for the benefit of the group *and* it does not disclose any current eating disorder symptoms. Allow participants to share as much as is comfortable. After participants have shared, summarize what you heard and model encouragement and hope.

---

20 I ordered it this way so that clients have already been thinking about the different ways hunger can manifest. I think that makes it easier to then consider what could disrupt that attunement. In *The Intuitive Eating Workbook*, self-care is presented before exploration of hunger. Adjust the order as you see fit.

Step 1: Between-Session Exercises Debriefing

There were three potential between-session exercises for the previous week: **How Has Micromanaging My Eating Affected My Life? If Reframing Thoughts with Self-Compassion**, and **Letting Go of the Tools of Dieting**. Check in on how the exercises you assigned went. Did clients have any trouble completing them? How helpful were they? Did any exercises *not* resonate? Debriefing each exercise informs the feedback and support you offer now and going forward.

If during this debriefing you realize your client still has skepticism about dieting being harmful, or is unsure whether the intuitive eating approach is right for them, validate and normalize those feelings. Ambivalence is totally normal and understandable at this stage. Meet clients where they are.

Step 2: Explore the What and Why of Hunger

The first task of the session is to introduce hunger: what it is and why we feel it. Within diet culture, the importance of hunger is so diminished that people often don't even pause to consider its utility. Many of us have so deeply internalized the idea that we must rely on rules to dictate our eating that we forget (or are unaware) that our bodies have inborn regulatory systems designed to help us know when, what, and how much to eat. Linking the function of hunger to other bodily cues can help clients begin to see hunger as necessary and useful instead of bothersome or guilt-inducing.

Many things can affect whether and how we experience our hunger cues, including food insecurity, regular restriction or eating past fullness, exercise, certain medical conditions and treatments, and neurodiversity such as autism and ADHD. For instance, when hunger consistently goes unheeded, whether intentionally or not, the body can adapt by suppressing these signals. However, when food becomes available again, the body often takes over, which can result in bingeing. Further, the messages we get about how much, what, and when we should eat from social media, family, friends, and healthcare providers can make the process of tuning in to our bodies confusing, and we might not trust that what we're feeling is truly hunger.

Here's an exercise you can use to help clients begin to see hunger as an important biological cue. You can skip it if you perceive your client already thinks about hunger in this way, or if de-emphasizing eating according to hunger is clinically indicated with your client.

EXERCISE: Hunger Is Just Another Cue

1. **What do you notice happens in your body when you need to sleep?**
    Does your client notice they have the urge to lie down? Get in bed? Do they start yawning? Is it harder to pay attention to what they are doing?

2. **What about when you're too hot or too cold? How does your body let you know it needs your help regulating your temperature?**

   Do they start to sweat, or shiver? Do they add or remove clothing? Do they notice they have a restless feeling they can't easily ignore until they address the situation?

3. **When you notice you need to go to the bathroom, what do you do?**

   This will likely generate laughs, but roll with it! Clients may point out there are times they cannot use the restroom when they need to, like during a timed test or while on an airplane. However, they likely aren't questioning whether they actually need to go, nor are they likely trying to avoid going unless there's a genuine need to wait.

4. **What happens if you ignore these cues? Let's say that you need to go to the bathroom, but you keep trying to ignore the need. Will it eventually go away?**

   The point of this is to help them see that, eventually, the body will get its needs met. When we need to go to the bathroom, eventually we'll go, one way or another. When we need to sleep, eventually we cannot fight the urge and we will fall asleep. Similarly, if we restrict our food or try to ignore hunger for long enough, our bodies will almost always take over (provided food is available). Of course, there are some exceptions. However, the goal is to show clients that responding to periods of restriction with bingeing or loss-of-control eating is *not* a failure or a lack of willpower. Rather, this reaction reflects their bodies doing their best to protect them and survive!

If this exercise resonates with your client, it may be therapeutic to continue to unpack these points. For instance, how does viewing hunger as important biological communication differ from how they have viewed hunger before? What is it like to think about hunger in this way?

Step 3: Body-Cue Awareness

Although your client should now be oriented to *why* we experience hunger, they likely will still struggle to identify whether what they're feeling is *truly* hunger. To some degree, this is a normal part of the human experience—there are still times I'm not 100-percent sure if I'm hungry or just tired! The goal is not to aim for perfection, but instead to help clients cultivate better attunement to their internal cues. I find it's useful to have a term you can use to differentiate true physical hunger from other "hungry" sensations we may have (e.g., emotions, thoughts). Like Tribole and Resch (2017), I use "biological hunger," but pick whatever you think will resonate with your client.

It's common, and understandable, to view hunger as a negative experience. We sometimes feel we need to fight it off, avoid it, or ignore it. It's also common to approach eating like a simple logic problem. Clients might think, "I just ate—how can I already be hungry?" But *many* things

Session 2: Honoring Your Hunger

can lead us to experience true biological hunger again shortly after eating, and if we try to suppress or ignore those cues, we disrupt any trust we've developed with our bodies. As Tribole and Resch note in *The Intuitive Eating Workbook* (2017), chronic or recurrent food deprivation is traumatic. It won't be easy and it won't happen overnight, but the more you can help clients use their body's signals versus their thoughts to guide their eating, the more they will heal. The goal of this session is to help clients get in touch with and begin honoring their cues to ultimately reestablish trust with their body.

Step 4: How Does Your Hunger Speak to You?

Because hunger is often represented as a "rumbling" or "empty" feeling in the stomach, people aren't always aware of other ways hunger might show up in their bodies. Recognizing other signs of hunger can help your client reinforce hunger as an adaptive, even savvy, biological cue. For instance, hunger often results in increased thoughts about food and attentional bias toward food cues. The body is trying to nudge us to hop on opportunities to receive nourishment! If your client doesn't tend to experience hunger in the expected ways, they may ignore different signs of hunger until it reaches a primal level.

The next exercise is aimed at exploring the various ways our bodies let us know we need nourishment, so clients can start identifying how *their* bodies communicate hunger. If during this exercise you sense any frustration in your client, be sure to normalize that! It can be confusing to identify the communication we're receiving from our bodies and distinguish it from the messages we've absorbed about bodies, food, and eating. As always, I encourage patience and curiosity; learning and doing intuitive eating is a process, *not* a destination. In a group setting, I like to emphasize that there is no right or wrong way to experience hunger. If someone communicates that their body expresses hunger in unique ways, that's OK. Similarly, if someone in the group has greater access to their hunger cues, it isn't "better" somehow, just different.

EXERCISE: Discovering Hunger

1. **What do you feel in your stomach when you're hungry?**

    Clients may feel rumbling, churning, or emptiness. Some won't feel anything in their stomachs, which is also normal.

2. **What about in your head?**

    Common cognitive manifestations of hunger include feeling light-headed or foggy, struggling to focus, and having increased thoughts about food.

3. **What happens to your mood when you need to eat, or when it's been a long time since you've eaten?**

    Irritability ("hanger") is a common mood state that signals hunger. Clients may also experience apathy, sadness, increased anxiety, or feel more tense or on edge.

4. **Any other physical signs you notice?**

    Clients might notice low energy, sleepiness, or lethargy. They may get headaches. At its extreme, hunger can result in dizziness, shakiness, cold intolerance, and other symptoms of hypoglycemia.

At this point, you can process what your client has learned about their own signs of hunger. Is it possible they're missing more subtle signs of hunger? For clients that often don't realize they're hungry until it's extreme, are their bodies giving any other signs earlier?

With these insights generated, orient clients to the **Hunger Rating Scale**. The purpose of this scale is to illustrate the spectrum of hunger experiences and provide clients with a guide they can use in their own hunger discovery over the next week. The scale goes from 0, painfully hungry, to 10, painfully full, and each level is accompanied by a description. "Hunger quality" refers to whether the experience of hunger is pleasant, unpleasant, or just neutral. Primal hunger can be unpleasant because it's extreme and is often accompanied by *other* unpleasant sensations, like irritability or fatigue. Conversely, emerging hunger may be pleasant, possibly accompanied by some excitement about eating, especially when we know eating is imminent.

Over the next week, you want your client to practice observing and describing their hunger. With your client, arrive at a goal that feels feasible. I often ask clients to choose two or three days in which they can note the timing and locations of their meals and snacks and rate their hunger (both level and quality) before and after they eat on the **Hunger Discovery Log**. If entire days are not possible, clients can choose two or three meals or snacks over the course of the week.

If clients experience aversion to the sensations of hunger or fullness, you may want to skip rating hunger quality. Not everyone finds hunger or fullness pleasant, so rating the quality could be more harmful than beneficial. Make sure your client understands that you don't want them tracking calories, macros, or anything similar. The goal is to notice patterns and trends, such as common times of day when they are especially hungry *or* less connected to their hunger signals. The handout has space for their reflections that you can review in the session debriefing next week.

Step 5: Distinguishing Hunger Cues from Thoughts and Other Inputs

Although your client has some tools now to explore how their body communicates hunger, experiencing hunger can still be confusing. This is especially true when hunger has become so laden with meaning that it no longer represents a neutral biological signal but instead evokes guilt or shame. Hunger presents itself in many different ways, making it challenging to distinguish biological hunger from other states like tiredness. Further, we're surrounded by competing messages about eating and food, like seeing an advertisement promoting a weight loss company immediately followed by one promoting fast food. These factors lead us to become cognitive instead of intuitive about hunger, questioning whether we're *truly* hungry.

There are many reasons a person may need more food than usual. Maybe the day before they were more active or ate less than usual. Maybe they had a lighter meal, or ate foods that were less

Session 2: Honoring Your Hunger

satisfying, or had minimal fat or protein. Maybe they're experiencing normal hormonal fluctuations. Maybe it's just a hungrier day! Our bodies don't work according to perfect math equations. Some days we just need more! Sometimes hunger strikes at inconvenient times, and sometimes we won't be able to honor it right away. But most people have days when they're extra tired for no apparent reason and they probably aren't second guessing that!

The **Mind, Body Cue, or Self-Care** worksheet is intended to help clients distinguish among thoughts, body cues, and deficits in self-care. If you're lengthening treatment, I suggest working through the worksheet together in session. Otherwise your client can complete it between sessions.

At this stage of intuitive eating, it's common to overthink hunger. You do want to help your client learn to distinguish among body cues, thoughts, and emotions. However, the goal is *not* to encourage mental gymnastics every time your client experiences an urge for food. Be on the lookout for overthinking, and compassionately redirect. Let clients know that, when in doubt, they can eat! If they realize later that they weren't biologically hungry, that's good information to incorporate in the future.

Step 6: What Gets in the Way of Hunger?

Self-care has taken on new meaning in recent years. In media, it's often depicted as indulgence in bubble baths and manicures (no shade intended!). It's really about getting basic needs met. Some needs, like food, shelter, and security, are universal (Tay & Diener, 2011). Others, such as love, respect, and autonomy, also appear to be important to well-being, though their degree of importance varies by culture. When one or more of these core needs is not met, we struggle to adapt to our circumstances, maintain our mental health, meet our responsibilities, and show up for people in our lives.

When our level of self-care is low, our connection with our hunger cues can be disrupted. During graduate school, I taught a course on stress and its management. One of the first topics we covered was the fight-or-flight response, and what happens when our stress systems are repeatedly or chronically activated. I can't tell you how many lightbulbs went on in the room when we covered this content—connecting students' lived experiences with the physiology of the stress response. In the face of stress, our bodies have many responses that prepare us to fight, flee, or freeze. Blood flow is diverted toward our extremities, where it's needed, and away from our digestive systems. A consequence of *chronic* stress, however, is that it conditions us to feel less connected to our hunger cues. Our bodies, including the very useful fight-or-flight response, were not designed to endure the levels of chronic stress most of us encounter; some of us endure crushingly high levels. Therefore, adequate provision of self-care is fundamental to intuitive eating, and requires priority from us as clinicians. If a client has inadequate access to food, for instance, I focus on addressing that before I ever think about counseling them to eat when hungry. Some clients may see self-care as a luxury, or selfish. Indeed, it can come across as highly individualistic, which conflicts with some clients' values. To these clients I say, you can't pour from an empty cup. Ensuring their basic needs are taken care of helps *them* feel better so they can be a kinder, more patient parent, friend, sibling, child, or partner.

There is a **Self-Care Assessment** available (refer to it differently if the term "self-care" isn't preferred). Adapted from *The Intuitive Eating Workbook* (Tribole & Resch, 2017), this worksheet names several categories of needs (e.g., physical, social) associated with those circumstances that promote attunement and those that disrupt it. In session, have your client spend a little time looking it over and beginning to identify their strengths in self-care—what are they currently doing well? These could be categories (e.g., they prioritize their relationships) or individual actions or habits (e.g., meditating daily for five minutes). Are there areas or items they might want to work on or prioritize more?

I recommend picking one thing (and not more than two!) they can do in the week between sessions in the interest of self-care. They may want to prioritize more sleep during the week, drink less alcohol, or schedule relaxation time. Many people (myself included!) pick up their phone and start scrolling absentmindedly, which can feel guilt-inducing if you have tasks to accomplish. Clients might choose to notice when this happens, and practice making other choices, like disabling certain apps during the day and scheduling 30 minutes to watch a TV show or TikTok videos. When relaxation is *intentional,* it can alleviate guilt. If your client wishes, help them set a realistic goal, get concrete about how they'll achieve it, and consider what could get in the way.

Step 7: Between-Session Exercises and Closing

There's a lot of content in this session! In the following week, your client can focus on getting to know their hunger by tracking it on the **Hunger Discovery Log** using the **Hunger Rating Scale**. Again, I recommend guiding clients to pick a reasonable goal here—something like tracking for two or three days or tracking a few meals or snacks. Guide them to pick days or eating occasions when they'll have time and resources to pause and take notes.

Your client will pick one area of self-care to work on this week. The **Self-Care Log** provides space to track progress and reflect on any changes.

Closing

As always, close out the session by asking your client what hit home from the session or what will stick with them through the week. I like to reciprocate, modeling that I'm genuinely interested in their well-being and that I'm also always learning and growing.

Lengthening the Session

If time and resources permit, this session can be expanded into two. Lengthening this session may be especially useful if your client:

- Feels particularly disconnected from their hunger cues or struggles to identify ways they experience hunger
- Has a history of an eating disorder
- Has a history of food insecurity
- Experiences considerable barriers to self-care
- Associates hunger with guilt

To lengthen this session, I suggest:

- Spending the first session on Steps 2 through 4: the why and how of hunger.
- Spending the second session on Steps 5 and 6: sorting out hunger cues and identifying barriers to experiencing them.

Shortening the Session

For clients with diminished interoceptive awareness due to medical conditions, autism, or ADHD, you may want to focus less on getting to know biological hunger. You may perceive it would be more useful for your client to identify less-obvious signs of hunger, like cloudy thinking or irritability.

Rather than making **How Does Your Hunger Speak to You?** an interactive activity, you might instead list the various physical and cognitive signs of hunger and ask which resonate for them. You can spend less time on **Mind, Body Cue, or Self-Care** and provide that material in handout form, noting that diet culture can lead us to overthink and question our hunger.

What is essential to cover in this session in my view are: (1) *why* we experience hunger (helping to cast it as a neutral biological cue), and (2) the importance of self-care.

CHAPTER 6

Session 3: Finding Peace with Food

Session Outline

Step 1: Between-Session Exercises Debriefing

 Hunger Discovery Log

 Hunger Rating Scale

 Self-Care Log

Step 2: Overview of Finding Peace with Food

 Exercise: Exploring the Bounds Around Your Eating

 Handout: Food and Exercise Rules

Step 3: Habituation

 Exercise: Habituation Dissonance

 Exercise: Habituation or Graduated Exposure

 Optional Exercise: Common Habituation Fears

Step 4: Between-Session Exercises and Closing

 Food and Exercise Rules

 Habituation or Graduated Exposure

Materials

Food and Exercise Rules

Habituation or Graduated Exposure

Session Aim

Principle three, Make Peace with Food, is often understood as being about letting go of non-medically necessary rules around food, eating, and exercise. These may include restrictions about how much one eats (e.g., calories, macros), when one eats (e.g., intermittent fasting), or what one eats (e.g., carbs). Your client may have similar rules about the type, duration, or frequency of exercise they do.

I take a broader perspective of finding peace with food. In my view, this principle is about the bounds a person has created around their eating, either intentionally or unintentionally, and whether these bounds have more costs than benefits. I conceptualize this principle this way because I think you'll work with clients whose bounds may not look like traditional dieting. For instance, I've worked with a client who had a phobia of eating in public. This fear wasn't related to anti-fat bias or concern about others seeing (and judging) what they were eating. However, this phobia became so obstructive in their life that it interfered with relationships, school, work, and adequate nourishment. For this client, making peace with food involved exploring the nature and origin of their fear and then incorporating graduated exposure exercises. Ultimately, they progressed to eating in front of others, and began to generalize this behavior across settings and situations, resulting in considerable relief and quality-of-life improvement. All this is to say that the aim of this session is to explore (1) the bounds clients have around their eating and exercise, (2) costs and benefits of these bounds, and (3) ways to reduce or remove any bounds causing more distress than benefit.

Additional Considerations and Potential Adaptations

Food rules often come from a genuine desire to be "healthy" or take care of oneself. Sometimes they come from a desire to change one's body. There are many factors potentially contributing to the food-related beliefs and rules people hold and follow. For instance, if someone has had experiences with cancer or other serious illness, they're likely receiving messages about the role of foods in disease risk. They may have read books on dietary approaches purported to cure disease or prevent recurrence. Although people may undertake dietary changes to promote health and healing and prevent progression or recurrence, these rules can become obsessive and rigid. People may be trying to control what is controllable, and their behaviors can lapse into orthorexia or other disordered patterns. Rather than promoting health, these patterns of behavior can begin to harm health.

If a person realizes their gender doesn't align with their sex-at-birth, they may turn to dietary and exercise rules to delay puberty, build muscle, or reduce curves. Someone in a larger body might try intermittent fasting or keto, whether due to recommendations from their healthcare providers or to try to feel safer in a world that pathologizes and judges their body size. So, although food and exercise rules may have the intended result of body modification, the reasons are not always so simple as desiring thinness or muscularity. Often, the motivation is far more nuanced.

As you work with this principle, make sure you're listening to your client's story and not imposing your own assumptions. Avoid the temptation to oversimplify motivations or dismiss how dietary rules may serve to help clients feel safe in the world, or simply survive. This session's goal is to get your client thinking about the rules they follow and to start to analyze the cost-benefit ratio. This discussion could also elucidate other supports your client needs. If they are dealing with acute or chronic illness, gender dysphoria, body dysmorphia, obsessive-compulsive disorder, or other health concerns, additional supports or referrals may be needed.

Finally, seek out expert guidelines before undertaking this work with neurodivergent clients.[21] Some of this session's content may need to be modified. For instance, autistic people often eat a restricted range of foods due to sensory processing differences, may have differences in their integration of interoceptive cues, and do not habituate in the same way as neurotypical people. The idea is to work with neurodivergent people's strengths and needs, not against them.

What to Expect from This Session

Reactions to this session can be mixed. It can be immensely therapeutic for clients to learn that deprivation actually drives out-of-control feelings around food. Yet, change is scary. Your client has rules around food for a reason, even if these rules are ultimately causing more harm than good. Systematically and intentionally breaking these rules may evoke fear and won't be easy. There may be some reluctance or ambivalence. That's OK! You can validate and normalize those feelings *and* work with clients to begin letting go of the rules no longer serving them at a pace that feels manageable.

The possibility of psychological reactance is particularly relevant in this session: if clients feel their autonomy is threatened, they may want to cling even tighter to their rules. You may feel a sense of urgency to help them let go of their food rules, especially if it's clear they're causing harm. But clients are in the driver's seat, and it's far better to plant seeds than shut someone down entirely. Honor your client's independence while encouraging them to consider what a life free of their food rules might look like.

---

21   An excellent resource when working with neurodivergent people with disordered eating is found at https://nedc.com.au/assets/NEDC-Publications/Eating-Disorders-and-Neurodivergence-A-Stepped-Care-Approach.pdf.

Session 3: Finding Peace with Food

> ## Considerations for Group Interventions
>
> This session can be both tricky and particularly fruitful with a group. I provide an alternate group version of the first exercise, **Exploring the Bounds Around Your Eating**. While in individual sessions, you'll explore the specific bounds your client has around eating or exercise, in group settings, sharing individual beliefs or behaviors can be triggering for other members. This is especially true when with behaviors (e.g., restriction) that are valued in society and with behaviors that are judged (e.g., bingeing). Therefore, the group exercise is modified to avoid creating a triggering and ultimately harmful dynamic. Nevertheless, I find the discussion around the potential consequences of food rules particularly fruitful in a group environment, as members help generate insights for each other.
>
> For the **Habituation** exercise, be mindful of group dynamics when considering whether to have participants share their specific plans. The benefit of sharing specifics is reciprocal feedback and support between group members. For instance, a group member once shared they wanted to eat the yogurt offered at the dining hall but avoided it due to the sugar content. Yogurt was a great pick for this person's habituation exercise because it was a food they wanted but *voluntarily* avoided. The group helped this person come up with a plan to try yogurt three times that week when eating with their roommate; the following week, the group cheered their efforts to reintroduce the food.
>
> Nevertheless, there is the risk of triggering social comparisons in group (e.g., "I'm not scared of yogurt. Should I be?"). Such comparisons are great fodder to acknowledge and discuss as a group (e.g., "Hm, I wonder why restricting certain foods would be enviable"). Still, if you have several group members with eating disorder histories, you may want to guide the discussion away from comparison. Instead, group members might share that they're going to try eating a food they fear without naming the food, or that they're going to try to confront a feared eating situation (e.g., eating in front of someone).

Step 1: Between-Session Exercises Debriefing

In the previous session, the client was instructed to track their hunger on the **Hunger Discovery Log** using the **Hunger Rating Scale**, and to identify one specific self-care improvement goal. As you're reviewing the **Hunger Discovery Log**, reflect on any trends you and your client are observing. For instance, did they notice there are specific times of day when they're more or less hungry? People may undereat earlier in the day, which can set them up to eat past fullness later in the day. Eating past fullness is almost always shame-generating, but it makes sense in the context of undernourishment. Be alert to opportunities, like this, to provide context and compassion. Reviewing this exercise can also highlight how accessible your client's hunger cues feel to them. If they're feeling pretty numb to hunger, recommend regular, consistent eating every three to four waking hours, and no more than six when possible. Explore with your client how hunger is *not* a prerequisite to eating and that nourishment is one way they can take care of themselves.

Some clients may still be struggling to differentiate between biological hunger and thoughts. For instance, they may head to the fridge an hour after dinner, then stop because they think, "I can't be hungry. I just ate. I must be bored." Maybe so. But explore how this is a time to get curious: "I just ate" is a thought; when they check in with their *body*, what do they notice? Are they experiencing any other signs of biological hunger? If they wait ten minutes, do their thoughts keep gravitating back to food?

With the **Self-Care Log**, celebrate wins and troubleshoot barriers and challenges. Sometimes prioritizing self-care is difficult because of low self-compassion. A client may not feel they're *worthy* of compassion or care, and may even fear self-compassion or see it as a barrier to their goals. For clients with low self-compassion or high self-criticism, you'll likely want to continue integrating compassion-focused exercises. You can continue practicing thought reframing, but might also add expressive writing or other activities that target self-compassion directly.

Step 2: Overview of Finding Peace with Food

Finding peace with food is about moving away from non-medically necessary food rules that cause more harm than benefit.[22] Although such rules often keep people stuck in harmful patterns, clients are likely following the rules because they're trying to take care of themselves.[23] If we hear repeatedly that sugar is inflammatory and carcinogenic, it makes sense to want to reduce or omit sugar. However, viewing sugar as "off-limits" and "bad" doesn't reduce its appeal. Rather, the idea that we can't have sugar makes it *more* appealing, and our thoughts about it are likely to increase, not decrease. Further, when something is restricted and we don't have the opportunity to habituate to it, it will continue to evoke the same (or even a stronger) reaction each time it's encountered. It's no wonder restriction can make us feel out of control! If a person is avoiding sugar, their cravings are likely to increase (as may their obsessive thoughts about sugar), and they're more likely to notice when sugar is around. Avoiding sugar will begin to require extraordinary levels of intention and effort. This could mean that many of such a client's resources are subsumed by focusing on sugar (a focus that may be at odds with their values). It could also mean that at some point this client binges on a food high in added sugars. Either way, their hypothesis

---

22 Throughout this chapter I refer to "food rules" as a shorthand for rules, guidelines, or limits around eating or activity that aren't medically necessary, guided by religious principles, or made for ethical reasons (e.g., vegetarianism).

23 For some, disordered eating behaviors can be a form of self-harm. If low self-compassion or fears of self-compassion are barriers to progress, you may want to integrate self-compassion-focused exercises early in treatment to increase engagement.

is seemingly confirmed. Experiencing obsessive thoughts about and cravings for sugar will make their belief that sugar is addictive feel very true. Similarly, if once a person eats sugar, they "lose control," their belief that they can't control themselves around sugar is strengthened. It can be powerful to help clients see this in another way. Explore: if they *are* losing control around a food or having obsessive thoughts and strong cravings, could something else be going on? If they had unconditional permission to eat those foods, what might happen?

Clearly, how you introduce and approach this principle will depend on the concerns of your client or group. For a client with an eating-related phobia, I deemphasized dieting and focused on understanding the fear-avoidance cycle and how the bounds that had emerged around their eating were impacting their life more broadly. This exploration helped them identify a gap between the life they were living and the one they wanted, which generated enough dissonance to motivate change.

EXERCISE: Exploring the Bounds Around Your Eating

In our clinical training, we learn that helping clients arrive at insights on their own is much more powerful than telling them what to do (especially because *they* are the experts of their experience). So, to get started with the principle of finding peace with food, I recommend an interactive activity wherein you guide your client to identify the bounds they have around their eating and exercise, and explore how these affect their lives more broadly. If they realize they have boundaries or rules that are hurting more than helping, you can ask them to envision their life without them. I provide two versions of this activity, one for individual sessions and one for groups.

Throughout this exercise, you want to reinforce that the bounds your client has around their eating or activity are often coming from a well-intentioned place. Many folks start a diet or lifestyle change because of the perceived health benefits. They may have realized they don't feel good in their bodies and wanted to try something they heard might help them feel better. Intuitive eating *absolutely* supports eating nutritious foods and thinking about how foods feel in your body. This exercise helps clients get curious about whether the bounds they have around eating are working for them, and what life could be like without them.

At the beginning of the exercise, provide the **Food and Exercise Rules** handout to guide discussion. Questions for discussion appear below; you don't have to ask every question; rather, let the conversation flow naturally, provided it stays productive. I like to introduce the activity with a comment like this:

> Many people have bounds around their eating and exercise. These could include rules around the frequency, amount, or type of food they can consume or exercise they should complete. Or the bounds could involve avoidance of certain foods or eating situations. These bounds can feel important because they're to improve health or create a sense of safety. But sometimes they start to harm more than help.

Individual Sessions

1. **What are some rules or limits around food, eating, or exercise you've had in the past or currently have?**

    Your client can review the **Food and Exercise Rules** handout to jog their thinking. Feel free to recall things they've mentioned if they're struggling to think of examples.

2. **Think about a couple of rules or limits that have felt particularly powerful in your life. What motivated you to create these bounds? What was or is the intended result?**

    What was your client hoping they'd gain by following these rules? *Or* what were they afraid would happen if they *didn't* follow them? Try to tease out what they stand to gain *or* lose.

3. **What happens if you step outside the bounds or break a rule?**

    For someone who's restricting, do they eat the off-limits food with a sense of loss of control? Do they vow to never eat the food again? Do they notice that the binge sets off a cycle of continued bingeing?

    Some people may not break or even relax their rules; for instance, if someone has a food-related phobia, they may go to serious lengths to avoid the feared situation. In these cases, you might ask, "What are you worried would happen if you violated this rule?"

4. **What effects do these bounds or rules have on your life?**

    The handout has space for the client to document the effects of the chosen bounds on their mood, resources (time and money), social life, work or school, and future goals; add categories relevant to your client. If your client is struggling to identify effects (both positive and negative), you may highlight things you've heard from them in the past, gently, and with compassion.

    I often hear from people following keto or intermittent fasting that life can become much smaller. They no longer go to brunch on the weekends. They must bring their own food to restaurants and social gatherings. They risk offending family members if they don't eat the foods served. They may experience digestive discomfort, extreme hunger, irritability, cold intolerance, and more. Their cravings may intensify, or their thoughts about food become more obsessive. Their relationships may be harmed: they may stop dating, or struggle to concentrate at work or school. They may also observe some benefits: maybe they *do* feel physically a bit better, or less anxious or more comfortable. The key is to explore the relative weight of each cost and benefit: it's not just the *number* of pros versus cons, but their degree of importance and meaning for your client.

5. **Think of a rule that may cause more harm than good. Imagine you no longer need it and can let it go. If your life were free from this rule, what would be different?**

Imagining a life without these boundaries can generate both relief *and* fear. Again, boundaries are often created with good intentions. Letting them go may feel unsafe to your client, or they may feel their health would be at risk. You can tie this discussion back to any consequences your client identified. For instance, "You mentioned some of your friendships have suffered because you're not going out as much and are starting to avoid events where there will be food. Would that change if you no longer followed this rule?"

Optional Question For clients who are particularly fearful or reluctant about letting go of their food-related boundaries, I like to ask them to imagine someone close to them, or even to imagine themselves as children.

6. **Imagine your closest friend is going through the same thing. What would you want for them? What might you say to encourage them to take a step toward change?**

    People often find it easier to generate empathy for others—or even a younger version of themselves—than to show self-compassion.

After this exploration, summarize the discussion with your client. Let's say your client shared that intermittent fasting felt empowering when they were able to stick to it, and led to a little weight loss, which they liked. However, they realized they've begun to feel anxious when they're invited to brunch or parties where people will be drinking and snacking late into the evening. Additionally, they struggle to get work done in the morning during their fasting hours, and have been more irritable with their partner. You might reflect, "It sounds like you've noticed some changes from intermittent fasting that you like, but you're also noticing it's hard to sustain and is making work and relationships more challenging. The idea of a life where you don't have to restrict your eating to certain times of day is appealing, but you're also afraid of losing control. It sounds like you've never really given yourself unconditional permission to eat, but you would want that for your best friend. Does that sound right?"

Group Sessions

Remind group members that when we mention food rules, we mean rules about what, how much, and/or when to eat that are not driven by medical, religious, or ethical reasons.

1. **What are some food rules you've heard of people having?**

    Examples might include low sugar, low carbs, intermittent fasting, no eating after seven at night, no snacks, and so on.

2. **Some of you may have tried some of these things, or know people who have. When trying to follow these rules, do you notice any changes in your thoughts, emotions, or behaviors? How does it typically go?**

    Group members may notice a pattern of initial enthusiasm or motivation that wanes over time. Some may become more obsessive, rigid, and sensitive to perceived "failures." Some may become more withdrawn or moodier than usual. It's common for some to initially feel more empowered or confident, though this feeling is often vulnerable to perceived lapses.

3. **How much energy or time does it take to follow these rules?**

    Not all rules group members have will be mentally or emotionally taxing to follow. And if members have been following the rule(s) for a long time, they're likely on autopilot. In this case, it might be useful for them to consider how challenging it was at the beginning. What was their life like *before* these rules? Did they have more time or mental energy than they have now?

4. **How does following these rules affect your life? Do you notice any effects on your school or work, your relationships, or your physical or emotional health?**

    Often, there are costs to trying to follow food rules. Yet, because the consequences can accumulate incrementally, group members may not be fully aware of them. They may experience productivity or time management issues with work or school because their focus is affected. They may experience various challenges in their relationships. They may have less time for socializing, experience mood or libido changes, or try to avoid certain social situations involving food. Dieting can certainly affect physical health: people can experience increased gastrointestinal discomfort, fatigue, lightheadedness, or feeling foggy, and may face issues like anemia or irregular or absent menstrual cycles.

5. **What does it feel like when you break a food rule? What happens after?**

    Often food rules are set up as a system of pass or fail. What's worse, because we must eat multiple times every day, we're confronted with endless challenges to these rules. For instance, if you cut carbs, you're likely navigating multiple occasions to avoid carbs (or not) every day.

    After breaking a rule, people may become even more determined, setting rules that are more extreme. Or clients might find themselves in a cycle where they have let all their rules go and feel out of control, which also elicits distress.

6. **How sustainable are these rules? Do you believe people are usually able to stick to them?**

    Clients often think *they* are the problem, not the rules. You may want to reality-test that a bit: Given the ubiquity of diet and weight loss information and the oppressive presence of weight stigma, if it were easy to diet and lose weight, wouldn't everyone have accomplished it?

This week between sessions, you'll ask clients to take an inventory of the ways they micromanage their food, eating, and body image and then answer some reflection questions on the **Food and Exercise Rules** handout. Working on this between sessions gives clients more space and time to safely process what they're learning about their relationship with food rules and explore how such rules are and aren't serving them.

Session 3: Finding Peace with Food

Step 3: Habituation

This week, you'll ask your client to do a between-session exercise that's potentially quite challenging: relaxing, or breaking, one of the boundaries they have set around eating. This could mean reintroducing a feared or challenging food, eating at an off-limits time (e.g., after 9 p.m.), or confronting a challenging eating situation (e.g., eating in front of others). Some clients may be understandably reluctant to do this exercise; giving them information about habituation will provide helpful context. Essentially, habituation reflects getting so used to something that it no longer evokes a strong reaction. If someone becomes habituated to a food, it means they no longer experience intense fear or overwhelming cravings when it is presented. Habituation doesn't mean food is no longer enjoyable—it just has less power over one's emotions.

To further reinforce the concepts, you'll do an in-session exercise where your client encourages a friend to relax one of their food rules. If your client still has lingering concerns about doing the habituation exercise, I provide an optional in-session exercise below.

As mentioned, non-medically necessary food rules can have paradoxical effects. When something is deemed off-limits, the desire for it often becomes stronger, and rules and behaviors around it can become more extreme.

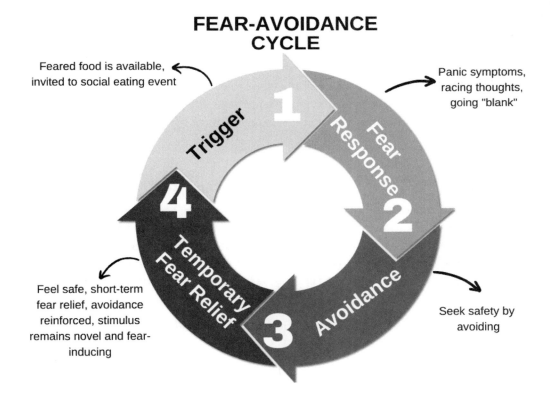

Put into food terms, imagine someone has decided to omit sugar from their diet because they have come to believe sugar is addictive and unhealthy. Thus, sugar is "dangerous," and they want to avoid it. However, there are two problems: (1) sugar is almost totally unavoidable, and (2) this person *really* likes many foods containing sugar. The more they attempt to avoid sugar, the more obsessive the thoughts about sugar become and the stronger the cravings get. Sugar has become a Big. Deal. Eventually, they're likely to break their rule. Because sugar is "off-limits," they're also more likely to eat it with a last supper mentality. Even as they eat it, they may be recommitting to avoiding it in the future. Since this is the last time, they may eat until they're uncomfortably full. These events further reinforce that sugar is dangerous; that they're out of control around it; and that they need to avoid it. They never habituate to sugar because it's off-limits, remaining dangerous and novel.

The pattern is usually different when one is limiting or avoiding certain foods for other reasons. If every time you eat apples, you experience uncomfortable gas and bloating, you may realize that apples don't agree with your body. Although you love apples, eating them is not worth the discomfort. In this scenario, apples are not coded as "bad," and eating them is probably not seen as a failure of willpower. You may miss apples, but you choose to eat other fruits that don't cause discomfort. It's also rare for patients to report bingeing on kale or quinoa, foods coded as "healthy." Foods that don't have the allure of danger are rarely off-limits; thus it's easier to eat them in satisfying quantities.

Making peace with food is about generating awareness of one's food rules and beginning to reintroduce previously feared or avoided foods. You'll want to discuss the concept of habituation with your client, and how restricting what, how much, or when one eats can have rebound effects. Having that context can decrease shame as your client realizes they're not actually out of control. The following exercise is designed to reinforce your client's understanding of habituation. If you're doing this in a group, you can make it into a role-play. Group members can pair off and take turns playing the role of someone with a food rule and the role of a friend encouraging them to let the food rule go. Alternatively, group leaders can role-play as the person with a food rule and let each group member contribute to encouraging them to relax their rule.

EXERCISE: Habituation Dissonance

Imagine one of your loved ones has a rule about what, how much, or when to eat. For instance, maybe your closest friend is trying to give up sugar. They've expressed to you that it's getting harder and their cravings for sugar are getting more intense. They've tried to eat fruit when they have a craving, but it rarely satisfies their urge. A couple of times they've ended up bingeing, which makes them feel out of control and like they failed. They confide that they think they may be addicted to sugar.

1. How would you explain the concept of habituation to this person?

2. **What would you say to encourage this person to try a habituation exercise with sugar?**

Note that some may have a genuine concern about whether the amount of sugar they're consuming is negatively affecting how they feel physically. However, if your client perceives sugar is *bad* and thinks they're bad for eating it, then sugar is likely to remain alluring and may even be subject to a cycle of deprivation and bingeing. Making peace with sugar so that it's emotionally neutral will set the stage for gentle nutrition later when they can begin considering how different foods make them feel physically.

This week, you'll ask your client to do a **Habituation** exercise or a **Graduated Exposure** exercise between sessions (they can document their progress on the accompanying handout). Details about these exercises follow.

Habituation

Help your client pick **one** rule (e.g., not eating until noon), feared or restricted food (e.g., ice cream, yogurt, chips), or eating situation (e.g., eating in front of people) to practice with this week. Collaborate to determine what is feasible and realistic: the aim is to practice eating this food, confronting the feared eating situation, or relaxing the rule **three times** this week (e.g., eating ice cream, eating in front of someone, or eating before noon).

Your client should plan what, when, and with whom. What will their goal be? When will they do it (specific days and times)? Will they involve a supportive person? It can help to practice eating a feared food, for instance, with someone they trust who can provide support during the exercise.

The food should be the exact same between trials. For instance, if it's ice cream, it should be the same kind each time. If the food changes, habituation will take longer. Generalizing across different flavors of ice cream can come later.

If practicing with a feared or restricted food, your client should not be too hungry before the trial. It's best if they have food in their system. If they're overly hungry, they're more likely to eat rapidly, eat past fullness, or feel a sense of loss of control. This may reinforce the fear or avoidance response.

Graduated Exposure

For clients with phobias related to food or eating, you may want to do a graduated exposure (aka systematic desensitization). Many online resources can provide an in-depth overview of the technique. Briefly, you and your client create an exposure hierarchy that involves listing feared situations from least to most distressing. For a client with a fear of eating around people, the first step involved ordering food on an app and having it delivered. A bit later in the hierarchy, they went into a fast-food restaurant, ordered food at the counter, and ate in the car. Gradually, they worked toward eating in the restaurant, first at an off-peak time and later when the restaurant was busy. After that, we moved to generalizing to other situations (e.g., eating at work). If your client is having trouble getting started on their own, I recommend doing exposures in-session.

If you perceive your client is *not* ready for exposure exercises, assess what might be coming up. Your client might need more time to process their food and eating-related beliefs (Session 4), or more support with coping (Session 6) or body image (Session 7). It's also possible these exercises are not right for your client.

OPTIONAL EXERCISE: Common Habituation Fears

If you notice your client or group seems a bit fearful of doing a habituation exercise, take some time to go through common fears and assumptions. Ask what fears are coming up for them. Here are some fears that have come up often in my work:

1. "Once I start eating [food], I won't stop."

2. "I don't trust myself around [food]."

    Some clients may feel these fears are well founded. They may have felt out of control around food in the past. Revisit the research that dietary restraint makes one more likely to eat past fullness because it makes foods more rewarding, makes one more likely to notice food cues in their environment, and increases the number and frequency of thoughts about food. Let them know that once people eat an off-limits food *without* giving themselves truly unconditional permission, they're more likely to vow to restrict that food again, which perpetuates the cycle. If your client has experienced a sense of loss of control when eating a specific food, ask: Were they giving themselves unconditional permission to eat that food?

3. "I don't know who I am without [food rule]."

    Sometimes, a client's identity gets enmeshed with their food rules. This is especially true for clients with current or past experiences of disordered eating and eating disorders. They may feel their food rules reflect who they are (e.g., disciplined, determined). Or they may feel their food rules are an important part of how their loved ones see them. If they leave their food rules behind, they may fear people in their life will see and treat them differently. Your client may not know who they are without these rules, and that can be understandably fear-inducing. Explore with your client whether the relative benefits of holding onto this sense of identity outweighs the consequences.

    I once had a client with a diagnosis of ARFID whose food limits were due to the aversive consequences of eating. This client had been weight-suppressed for so long that their body size had become a part of their identity. Their health was compromised and weight restoration was a critical goal; yet the idea of increasing their intake to the point of substantial weight restoration was scary. A clinical supervisor of mine once said we often prioritize destructive comfort over constructive discomfort. For this client, we had to work on developing other parts of their identity so that their body size was less central to their sense of self. In a weight stigma–saturated world, gaining weight was still understandably fear-inducing.

4. "I'll gain weight if I [behavior]."

    Fearing weight gain is not just a matter of vanity. For some, gaining weight could genuinely compromise their safety. Those who recover into larger bodies will face greater discrimination, and this can be compounded for those with other marginalized identities; for instance, Black women. Queer men who gain weight may encounter increased romantic rejection and stigma as their bodies diverge from their community's appearance standards. These are founded fears, and addressing them may require an individual cost/benefit analysis. Clients can be guided to ask: What does this body shape or size give me, and what does it cost me? What would I gain and lose if I stopped trying to micromanage my body size?

5. **"I need [behavior] for my mental health."**

    For some, eating and exercise behaviors may function to regulate affect or provide a sense of safety. For these and similar reasons, advocates call for a shift away from an abstinence-based view of disordered eating recovery and toward a harm-reduction approach: mitigating or reducing potential harms associated with risky behaviors, in order to improve quality of life, health, and overall functioning.[24] If your client is struggling to make changes because their behaviors are serving a self-regulatory function, you may want to move up the session on coping with emotions (Chapter 8). In that session, you can identify other ways your clients may be able to meet their emotional needs that are less risky or harmful. Additionally, your client does not need to change everything overnight. Meet them where they are.

Step 4: Between-Session Exercises and Closing

You have some options this week for between-session exercises. You'll ask all clients to engage in further reflection on the **Food and Exercise Rules** handout. Then, you'll assign either a **Habituation** or a **Graduated Exposure** worksheet depending on your client's concerns. Some clients may be ready to introduce a previously off-limits food or take a break from intermittent fasting, for instance. For these clients, you can jump into **Habituation**. If your client has food- or eating-related phobias or isn't quite ready for habituation, you may want to do a **Graduated Exposure** activity.

Closing

Close out by asking your client what from the session will stick with them through the week. As always, if something the client said resonated with you or if you were particularly struck by your client's vulnerability or insight, share that!

---

24   https://www.nationaleatingdisorders.org/blog/rethinking-healing-through-lens-harm-reduction.

Lengthening the Session

This can be a challenging session. When time permits, you may want to lengthen this session into two if your client:

- Has a history of an eating disorder

- Has a lengthy dieting history

- Has extensive or entrenched rules around eating or exercise

- Has a food- or eating-related phobia: you may want to continue practicing exposure exercises throughout treatment, even when moving onto other content (provided exposure is not contraindicated)

- Lives with or is close to people who are dieting

To lengthen this session into two, I suggest:

- Spending the first session on exploring the bounds around eating: if you're beginning habituation or exposures, start with something small in the first session. In the second session you can get into the theory behind habituation/exposure and make a detailed hierarchy.

- Spending the second session on habituation

Shortening the Session

For clients who have trauma histories or are neurodivergent, you may not want to do exposure or habituation. If your client doesn't have many bounds around their eating,[25] briefly introduce these concepts, as the information may become pertinent later in their life. However, you may not need to do habituation or exposures.

---

25 Assess these bounds carefully; some clients with binge eating, for example, may not realize that dietary restraint or restriction is actually maintaining their binge or emotional eating. Similarly, don't assume someone with a history of food insecurity or poverty-related deprivation is without bounds around their eating. Even after clients become food secure, binge eating may continue and could bring considerable distress. Check your clinical assumptions.

CHAPTER 7

Session 4: Challenging Thought Patterns

Session Outline

Step 1: Between-Session Exercise Debriefing

Habituation or Graduated Exposure

Step 2: Overview of Challenging the Food Police

Exercise: Exploring Food-Related Beliefs

Exercise: Evaluating Food-Related Beliefs

Step 3: Responding to Food-Related Comments

Exercise: Navigating Food-Related Conversations and Comments

Step 4: Between-Session Exercises and Closing

Personal and Family Food Rules

Responding to Food- and Eating-Related Comments

Materials

Personal and Family Food Rules

Responding to Food- and Eating-Related Comments

Session Aim

Even if clients aren't dieting, they've likely assimilated plenty of information about how to eat from their environments. When I was young, common messages I heard were that calories, fat, and sugar should be limited; desserts were unhealthy and indulgent; vegetables were the pinnacle of health; and eating after 8 p.m. was bad. Over time, eggs have fallen out of and back in to favor; carbs have taken on an almost villainous role; processed and packaged foods are portrayed as barely even consumable; and, of course, sugar is toxic. Adding to the confusion are dieting trends that starkly contradict each other. As of this writing, two trending diets are the carnivore diet, limiting you to only animal-based foods, and plant-based diets, limiting you to only plant-based foods. Keto is heralded as a panacea for all sorts of issues beyond the seizure disorders it was developed for, and intermittent fasting is touted as boosting longevity and mental clarity. There are also articles about keto increasing risk for cardiovascular disease and intermittent fasting leading to amenorrhea and reduced bone density. No wonder eating is so contentious and confusing—no matter how you eat, *someone* will think you're doing it wrong.

Even the idea that there is any one best diet for all of humankind is absurd. Humans evolved in many different regions and climates, where nutrition needs and food availability varied. Inuit populations historically consumed a lipid-rich diet, due in part to the Arctic climate and availability of foods high in fat (Fumagalli et al., 2015). Kenyan dietary patterns often reflect about 70 percent carbohydrate consumption, much of it teff and other grains, similarly due to crop availability and climate (Hansen et al., 2011). Bodies adapt accordingly; for instance, there is evidence of a genetic mutation occurring more frequently among the Greenlandic Inuit that affects glucose uptake, likely evolving from a hypoglycemic diet (Moltke et al., 2014). Thus, it is extremely unlikely there is any one *right* way to eat.

The goal of this session is to help your client begin disentangling their own food- and body image–related beliefs, including where they came from and whether they still hold up. Your client will also learn how to challenge, reframe, and defuse from (i.e., separate from) beliefs that are no longer working for them. (These cognitive restructuring and defusion skills are useful in *all* areas of life—not just eating!)

What to Expect from This Session

Our beliefs feel highly personal. Even if beliefs don't hold up to scrutiny, it can feel like an attack or a loss to have them threatened. Although we risk reactance in most of the sessions outlined in this manual, the risk is particularly high in this session. So, as always, keep your client's autonomy front and center: you're not telling them what to believe, but encouraging them to reflect on and get curious about the nature and outcomes of their beliefs.

We absorb a lot of information before we have fully developed our critical thinking skills. When exploring the origins of their beliefs, clients may feel protective of and hesitant to criticize their parents or family members. Most likely, their families were doing their best with the information they had; let your clients know this principle is not intended to criticize their loved ones. I designed the exercises in this chapter with care, so that clients can feel safe to explore and challenge their food-related beliefs. Still, it's important to keep these dynamics in mind throughout this session.

Additional Considerations and Potential Adaptations

The origins of each person's beliefs about food and bodies are complicated and interwoven. I find that a socioecological lens is useful in considering what influences our understanding of nutrition. For instance, public policy impacts what foods are available and to whom (e.g., through restrictions on which foods people can buy using public assistance funds). At the community level, cultural norms regarding appearance, body size, and feeding practices have profound influences on food choices. In some countries and cultures with high poverty, for instance, it's common for a larger body size to be seen as a sign of health. Also, in a context of poverty and food insecurity, wasting food is often discouraged, which can lead to pressure to clean one's plate. Institutions, families, and friends can reinforce these messages. For people who live amidst multiple cultures or whose identities are marginalized, these various messages can conflict, creating tension. People who immigrate to a country when they are young, for example, may experience competing pressures from the dominant culture and from their culture(s) of origin. All this is to say that your client's beliefs will almost always make sense within the broader context in which they developed. Knowing this should help you hold compassion as your client works to distinguish what they have absorbed from what they choose to embrace going forward.

Considerations for Group Interventions

This session's exercises are *great* for groups. The varied perspectives and experiences of group members generate excellent fodder for exploring and evaluating food-related beliefs and navigating unhelpful messages. Social comparisons can also occur when members are sharing and reframing food-related beliefs. For instance, one group member may share the belief that eating cheese is bad for you, and another member might feel shame because they've never questioned eating cheese. You can frame these and any other beliefs and experiences neutrally, as differences that clients can approach with curiosity.

Step 1: Between-Session Exercise Debriefing

In the previous session, clients began exploring the bounds they have around their eating and exercise. They were encouraged to spend time between sessions creating an inventory of these bounds and answering reflection questions. Check in on whether they had any additional insights after completing the inventory. Did they think of any other bounds they had around their eating or exercise? Reflect that they don't have to change everything overnight; rather, with more awareness they'll be able to decide what they do and don't want to change. Reinforce that awareness is a crucial first step!

Your client may have completed a **Habituation** or **Graduated Exposure** activity, which can be among the most challenging activities of the intervention. If your client didn't complete the exercise, explore that with openness and curiosity. What came up? Is it possible the goal needs revision? If you perceive your client may struggle to do this activity on their own initially, I recommend doing it together in a future session. Additionally, you may want to continue incorporating habituation or exposure activities into future weeks, *especially* if you created a fear hierarchy with clients in the last session. Some clients will be able to continue reincorporating previously off-limits foods and easing food rules on their own. Others will need more support and scaffolding.

Step 2: Overview of Challenging the Food Police

Throughout our lives, we absorb a ton of nutrition-related information, much of it before we have the cognitive tools to critically appraise the information. Within cultures obsessed with bodies and dieting, we take in *enormous* amounts of nutrition-related information. Your clients likely hold a lot of beliefs about food and eating, some of which may operate outside of their conscious awareness. To start this session, I do an exercise to bring food-related beliefs into conscious awareness. Once clients are aware of the beliefs they hold around food, they can begin to critically evaluate them. Because food and eating are so often described in moralistic terms, our food-related beliefs can feel deeply personal. It's hard to sort out what we believe from what we've been taught is true or "right." Therefore, the task is first to encourage nonjudgmental and curious exploration of both the origins and the outcomes of clients' food-related beliefs. Then, once your client has determined which beliefs they want to leave behind, you'll practice challenging and reframing them.

EXERCISE: Exploring Food-Related Beliefs

Using paper or a whiteboard, create three columns titled Beliefs, Origins, and Reframes. Ask your client or group members the following questions.

1. **Can you name some common beliefs about food, eating, or body image?**

    Your client may share beliefs they hold personally or that they have heard about online, through social media, or on podcasts; or they may share beliefs their families or friends hold. Some examples might be, "Processed foods are bad for you," "You shouldn't eat after 7 p.m.," or "Protein builds muscles."

    Write beliefs in the corresponding column. Try to get five to ten beliefs. It can be powerful for your client to visualize the many (and varied!) messages they've received about food, eating, and bodies.

Session 4: Challenging Thought Patterns

2. **Where do these beliefs come from?**

    Write the origins your client names alongside each belief; many will have several origins. Common origins include social media, online articles, parents, friends, TV, movies, influencers, and healthcare providers. Beliefs can also be cultural; for instance, some cultures or families may view eating what is served to be a sign of respect or of good manners. Or beliefs may originate from life experiences; for instance, families who experience food insecurity may have rules about not wasting food. Your client will likely realize these beliefs rarely have just *one* source. Rather, they are often transmitted at macro levels (institutions, mass media) and reinforced at micro levels (family, friends).

3. **Do any of the beliefs listed conflict with one another? Could it ever be feasible to follow all of them?**

    Could someone eat a keto *and* a plant-based diet? Avoid sugar entirely but also get plenty of vitamins and fiber from fruits and vegetables? For whom is it feasible to *never* eat processed foods? How avoidable are seed oils? Does your client see any signs of classism, racism, or ableism in the beliefs they have listed? Finally, if the rules *are* feasible, what would following all or most of them require in terms of time, money, skills, habits, relationships, social environment, and more?

EXERCISE: Evaluating Food-Related Beliefs

Ask your client to pick three to five identified beliefs to process further. Ideally these are the beliefs that your client holds most strongly or that are the most pervasive culturally. Generating awareness of these thoughts is the first step: because clients have been hearing these messages from so many sources for so long, their thoughts about food are likely automatic and are operating below their conscious awareness. So in this exercise we use techniques from acceptance and commitment therapy (ACT) and cognitive behavioral therapy (CBT) to defuse from and reframe unhelpful and inaccurate thoughts.

Before you start this exercise, define "automatic thoughts" for your client, explaining they are thoughts that pop up immediately in reaction to a trigger and that are often outside of conscious awareness. For example, thinking, "I'm so dumb!" immediately after dropping something.

1. **Let's start with the first belief. What automatic thoughts might come up related to that belief?**

    If your client needs help getting started, try placing the belief in context. If they have the belief that sugar is bad for you, what happens when they encounter sugar? For instance, if they are at dinner and everyone else decides to get dessert, what thoughts immediately come up? Some thoughts might be:

    - If I eat dessert, I'll lose control.
    - I don't want anyone to see me eating dessert.
    - If I eat dessert tonight, I need to work out harder tomorrow.

- Added sugars are bad for my health.
- I'm so weak for wanting to eat this dessert.

2. **Because automatic thoughts operate outside conscious awareness, we often react to them without evaluating them. When the thought is unhelpful or untrue, this can lead to trouble. We need to evaluate automatic thoughts, asking questions like, "Is this thought true? What evidence is there to support it?" If your thoughts have some truth to them, ask: "What is the context? Is this thought helpful? Could there be another way to see this?"**

Your client's experiences should be used to guide the evaluation of the thought. Thoughts could come from social media influencers, online articles, or well-intended advice from loved ones. Whatever the source, what does *your client's* experience tell them? Here are some examples:

Belief: If I eat dessert, I'll lose control.

Evaluating questions: What evidence supports this? When I've felt out of control around desserts in the past, did I have unconditional permission to eat *them*?

With this thought, it's important to consider if there's a history of food insecurity, which can make it harder to stop when full.

Belief: I don't want anyone to see me eating dessert.

Evaluating questions: What has happened in the past when I've eaten dessert with people? If people have judged me for eating dessert, does that make eating dessert wrong?

Belief: If I eat dessert tonight, I need to work out harder tomorrow.

Evaluating questions: What evidence is there that I need to earn food? How does it affect my relationship with movement when I use it to earn food? What would it be like if I were allowed to eat pleasurable food, independent of movement? What would it be like to engage in movement that wasn't tied to how "well" I had eaten?

Belief: Added sugars are bad for my health.

Evaluating questions: What health effects have I noticed from eating added sugars? How about from avoiding added sugars? What would it be like if I allowed myself to eat added sugars with attunement and intention?

Belief: I'm weak for wanting to eat certain desserts.

Evaluating questions: Would I view my friends as weak for wanting dessert? Is it weak to want to eat pleasurable foods? Does shaming myself for wanting dessert reduce my desire to eat it?

In the last example, you may want to note with your client that desserts are inherently rewarding for many reasons. They are associated with celebration and social bonding. They often contain sugar and fat, macronutrients that provide quick

Session 4: Challenging Thought Patterns

energy and aid satiety and satisfaction. It makes sense we would find foods that perform these functions pleasurable.

I don't advocate downplaying that foods vary in their nutrient density. Eating *only* desserts would rarely be health promoting (not always, though: milkshakes were all my grandfather would eat at the end of his life, and they were vital for providing nutrition and slowing his rate of decline). Yet, if a person has unconditional permission to eat desserts, they'd be free to eat desserts to satisfaction, without a last supper mentality. Because our bodies need an array of macro- and micronutrients, clients would likely notice their bodies operate best on a variety of foods—including, but not limited to, desserts. We'll dig more into this when we get to gentle nutrition (Session 9).

3. **Now, let's practice reframing thoughts or putting them into context**.

   After clients have evaluated their automatic thoughts, help them reframe these thoughts *or* put them into context. Here are some ways to do this based on the examples above.

   Thought: If I eat dessert, I'll lose control.

   Reframe: I feel out of control around desserts because I feel like I shouldn't have them. I haven't tried giving myself unconditional permission to eat desserts.

   Thought: I don't want anyone to see me eating dessert.

   Context: I'm scared to eat desserts in front of people because I've had people judge my food choices before.

   Related to the last example, the client may need to determine whether the person they're with is safe to eat dessert around. Explore possibilities with them. Is there anything they can say or do to protect their safety? If they're alone but in public, do they have the capacity to withstand potential judgment from strangers? If someone were to make a comment, how might they handle it?

   Thought: If I eat dessert tonight, I need to work out harder tomorrow.

   Reframe: Dessert doesn't have to be earned. I am allowed to enjoy pleasurable foods independent of exercise and move my body in ways that don't feel punishing.

   Thought: Added sugars are bad for my health.

   Reframe: Sugar is an important molecule our bodies use for energy. Restricting sugar has harmed my health more than eating it has.

   Thought: I'm so weak for wanting to eat this dessert.

   Reframe: Desserts are enjoyable and wanting to eat an enjoyable food is simply human.

The goal of the exercise is that your client has experience observing, evaluating, and reframing their thoughts. Reinforce that some thoughts can be evaluated and reframed, while others will be most amenable to nonjudgmental awareness of their context, and defusion.

For instance, regardless of how much progress we've made reducing anxiety, anxious thoughts will sometimes pop up. It can be cognitively taxing to reframe every single anxiety-inducing thought we have. When anxious or unhelpful thoughts pop up, the leaves on a stream exercise can be useful for cognitive defusion. Guide your client to visualize placing their thoughts onto leaves that are floating by on a stream, then simply watching them pass without following them downstream.

If a client remains fairly fused with their thought (e.g., believing sugar is toxic and thus avoiding sugar) and they don't wish to be, further evaluation and reframing will be useful; e.g., "Sugars are molecules our bodies use for energy. They're food. Eating them is a totally normal part of feeding my body." After the client does that work, those thoughts might still pop up, but either reframing will be more automatic or your client will be more easily able to allow the thoughts to pass without getting hooked.

Step 3: Responding to Food-Related Comments

It's huge for your client to start evaluating their food- and eating-related beliefs! Through this process, your client is establishing a new, and likely healthier, relationship with food and eating. Yet as your client changes, their environment may not. Although I have witnessed many clients keep strengthening their new relationship with food and eating—even to the extent of positively influencing the people around them—most live in environments that are full of threats to their newfound peace. Many family members and friends will still hold the food-related beliefs and follow the food rules clients are attempting to let go. And even if clients have strong support systems, most live in environments where food, eating, and body-related messages and comments are pervasive and unavoidable.

Across social situations, clients will encounter people making food- and eating-related comments, judging food choices, or reflecting shame for their own choices. Therefore, it can be helpful to practice how to respond to these comments. Context is important: what clients do or don't say will vary based on person, place, and time. I'll respond to a parent very differently than to a stranger. And I'll respond differently to my parent at a crowded family event than when we are one-on-one. Note also that this exercise is focused on food- and eating-related comments: we'll practice responding to body-related comments in Session 7 (Body Respect).

EXERCISE: Navigating Food-Related Conversations and Comments

In group settings, I do this exercise as a role-play. Leaders can play the role of a friend, family member, or stranger who is making a comment about food or eating. Group members can use what they've learned to respond and to help each other respond when someone gets stuck.

Session 4: Challenging Thought Patterns

Role-plays also work in individual sessions depending on your client's comfort. Alternatively, you can go through common comments and brainstorm responses together.

As always, be mindful of cultural and identity differences when doing this exercise. Some clients will experience diet talk and thinness pressures in their families or with friends; others may experience pressure to eat or to clean their plate. For some cultural groups, eating everything served is a sign of respect. Some clients may experience a combination of comments: pressure to clean their plate, even while weight- and body-related comments may be normative and thinness pressures are high. In a group setting, take care to be inclusive and provide space for everyone's experiences. You do *not* want the role-play exercise to only benefit the ethnic or racial majority group, or to include only material that speaks to some group members while excluding others.

Many clients will hesitate to be critical of their loved ones. It can help to note that most loved ones have the best intentions, and that the goal of this exercise is *not* to judge them. Rather, it's to help your client figure out how to navigate these conversations and protect their progress. (Although if your client needs to further process their reactions to loved ones' unhelpful comments, do so!)

1. **Do you worry that, as your relationship with food and eating changes, friends or family will judge your food choices?**

    Allow your client space to process this question. Their fears may indeed be reality based. It could feel interpersonally risky to eat in ways that align with their needs, but invite comments from loved ones.

2. **What are comments you've heard before, from a friend, family member, or stranger? Let's make a list!**

    In a group setting, encourage everyone to share. It's most helpful when responses represent the diverse experiences of your group. Comments can be ones clients hear regularly from family or friends, or they can come from tricky situations clients were unsure how to navigate.

3. **What are ways you could respond to these comments in the future?**

    Clients will use their own experiences, but here are some examples of comments and responses.

    - How are you still hungry? You just ate.

        My body is telling me it needs more food. I'm going to honor that.

    - You're really eating that?

        Yes, and it's delicious.

        Yes, food freedom tastes great.

    - I don't eat sugar. Sugar is addictive.

        It works best for me to not cut out entire food groups.

    - You're not going to eat the rest of that? But I made it for you.

        I really appreciate the love you put into this. Can I take some home to have later?

- I'm so full, I'm not going to eat until tomorrow.

    My body generally needs food every three to four hours, so I will still need to eat dinner.

- You shouldn't eat that, it's not healthy.

    For me, healthy eating is about not restricting myself from certain foods.

- Have more! We can't waste this food.

    This has been delicious. But I won't be able to enjoy it as much if I keep eating. Could I take what's left home?

- You should really watch what you eat, summer is coming!

    My body has the same needs in all the seasons!

It's important to note that sometimes the best thing to do is simply set boundaries or remove ourselves from the situation. We don't always have to speak up or advocate. When a stranger at a grocery store makes a comment, for instance, I sometimes have a reply ready. Sometimes, I grin uncomfortably and walk away. I might speak up if I perceive that I can use my privilege to have a positive influence; for example, talking to a medical provider who expressed weight bias.

There may be times when clients choose to eat in ways that don't align with their needs, whether that's eating a food they don't really want, eating past fullness, or choosing not to eat in situations that don't feel safe—this might be the safest course of action when loved ones or strangers won't respect your client's boundaries and needs. The goal is that your client makes their choice with intention and awareness.

Step 4: Between-Session Exercises and Closing

Your client gained valuable skills in this session! They practiced defusing from and reframing automatic thoughts and responding to negative food- and eating-related comments. Further practice will reinforce this learning and make these tools more readily accessible. During stressful experiences, clients will have more access to what they've practiced. So the between-session exercises this week are designed to give your clients opportunities to practice new ways of thinking about food and responding to food-related comments from others.

Between sessions, you'll ask your client to create a more detailed inventory of their personal and family food rules and beliefs (see the **Personal and Family Food Rules** handout). Then they'll critically evaluate these beliefs. Do they still feel true? How are they working for them? This critical evaluation will guide what your clients choose to *do* when related thoughts come up, whether that's cognitive defusion (i.e., observing thoughts with nonjudgmental awareness and allowing them to pass) or cognitive reframing (i.e., evaluating the truth and usefulness of automatic thoughts, and choosing alternate thoughts that better align with their values and goals).

For the other exercise, your client will continue to practice responding to food- and eating-related comments. Specifically, they'll log comments they hear throughout the week (whether directed at them or overheard) on the **Responding to Food- and Eating-Related Comments** handout, and brainstorm responses to those comments. They can note how they actually responded, and whether they want to respond differently in the future.

I recommend your client continue their habituation or exposure practice, if this was assigned. Depending on how this exercise went the previous week, you may choose to continue with the same food or situation or make a new goal.

Closing

As always, close out the session with something that resonated for you both.

Lengthening the Session

If your client has particularly entrenched food-related beliefs and experiences frequent unhelpful or negative thoughts about food or eating, you could easily spend the entire session on Step 2, Exploring and Evaluating Food-Related Beliefs. Similarly, if your client is exposed to many food- or eating-related comments in their life, or struggles responding to them, you could spend the entire session on Step 3, Responding to Food-Related Comments. In both cases, you would assign the relevant between-session exercise for that week. If your client is working on habituation or exposure, I recommend continuing those exercises each week.

Shortening the Session

You may choose to shorten this session if:

- This content is less salient for your client
- You have fewer sessions to work with

To collapse Sessions 3 and 4 into one session, you could:

- Provide an overview of Session 3 (Making Peace with Food), but omit the **Exploring the Bounds Around Your Eating** activity during session. This activity can be done as a between-session exercise.

- Give an overview of habituation and discuss common fears associated with letting go of food rules. Assign a **Habituation** or **Graduated Exposure** activity as a between-session exercise.

- Give an overview of strategies to challenge food-related beliefs and practice responding to food-related comments.

Alternatively, choose the content from this session that is most salient to your client. For instance, if your client is already adept at cognitive defusion and reframing, and is often exposed to harmful comments from others, you might focus more on responding to comments and less on exploring food-related beliefs.

CHAPTER 8

Session 5: Fullness and Satisfaction

Session Outline

Step 1: Between-Session Exercises Debriefing

   Personal and Family Food Rules

   Responding to Food- and Eating-Related Comments

Step 2: Overview of Feeling Your Fullness

   Exercise: How Do I Know When I'm Full?

   Handout: Hunger Rating Scale

Step 3: Barriers to Feeling and Honoring Fullness

   Exercise: Exploring Barriers to Fullness

   Optional Handouts: Distracted Eating, Clean Your Plate Club, Stopping When Full, Barriers to Fullness

Step 4: Discovering the Staying Power of Foods

   Macronutrients 101

   Exercise: Snack Pairing Experiment

   Handout: Snack Pairings

Step 5: Overview of the Satisfaction Factor

   But What Do I Want to Eat?

   Optional Exercise and Handout: Sensory Considerations

Step 6: Between-Session Exercises and Closing

   Getting to Know Your Fullness

   Hunger Rating Scale

   Barriers to Fullness

   Snack Pairings

   Optional: Sensory Considerations, Distracted Eating, Clean Your Plate Club, Stopping When Full

Materials

Hunger Rating Scale

Getting to Know Your Fullness

Distracted Eating (optional)

Clean Your Plate Club (optional)

Stopping When Full (optional)

Barriers to Fullness

Snack Pairings

Sensory Considerations (reference or optional activity)

Session Aim

In this session, you'll cover two interrelated principles: fullness and satisfaction. Just as our bodies provide signals to let us know we need nourishment, they nudge us when the need has been met, and we are full. However, it's rarely simple to notice and honor our fullness cues. Many folks feel disconnected from their fullness cues. Others notice when they're full but struggle to stop eating. Some find the sensation of fullness aversive, and avoid it. Further complicating matters is that fullness is complex—*many* factors affect our fullness levels, including but not limited to meal timing, amount eaten, types and combinations of foods, level of distraction, capacity for self-care, and emotional states.

Satisfaction is a crucial aspect of eating that is closely tied to fullness. Fullness signals that *enough* food has been eaten; satisfaction reflects a pleasurable sensation of contentment—that a person has eaten the foods their body needs and enjoys. Diets often promote eating in such a way that when people do experience fullness, it's both fleeting *and* unsatisfying. For instance, although eating a large bowl of (mostly) lettuce and drinking water may fill one's stomach, it's unlikely to be a *satisfying* meal because it's missing crucial macronutrients (fat, protein, non-fiber sources of carbohydrates). Cravings are also linked to satisfaction. Our bodies are smart, and they help guide us on not just *when* and *how much* to eat, but also on *what* to eat.

The aim of this session is to discuss the purpose of fullness, help your client explore how their body does and doesn't experience fullness, consider the various factors that affect fullness, and discuss the role of satisfaction in eating. You want to help your client gain better access to their fullness cues and eat in ways that honor their unique needs. Not all clients will be able to eat according to their hunger and fullness (e.g., clients in recovery from an eating disorder). However, this session can still help elucidate ways these clients can get their nutritional needs met even when fullness cues remain inaccessible or inconsistent.

Because two intuitive eating principles, Feel Your Fullness and Discover the Satisfaction Factor, are introduced in this session, there's a lot to cover. You can choose the activities and between-session exercises most salient to your client. If you have time, extending this session into two may be beneficial. See the end of the chapter for ideas on how to do so.

Additional Considerations and Potential Adaptations

Dieting, eating disorders, food insecurity, neurodivergence, and medical conditions can all affect people's access to and relationship with their fullness cues. Although it's useful for folks to have the information outlined in this session, not all clients should be encouraged to stop eating when they feel physically full. For instance, when someone is in recovery from a restrictive eating disorder (especially when working on weight restoration), early satiety is common. The same can be said for certain medical conditions that cause early satiety or decreased appetite. In these cases, working with a dietitian is crucial in finding ways to incorporate low-volume, nutrient-dense foods.

Session 5: Fullness and Satisfaction

For folks with lived experience of food insecurity, it can be challenging to stop at fullness. Clients may have learned to eat according to food availability rather than hunger and fullness. Although eating as much as possible when food is available is adaptive for survival, it can generate intense feelings of shame in an anti-fat, diet-obsessed culture. Additionally, neurodivergent folks may experience differences in their sensory integration, so relying on fullness cues may not be best for some neurodivergent clients.

This session has an activity designed to help people notice the subtle signs of fullness. It may help to explore whether your client is receiving signs, beyond physical fullness, that their needs for nourishment have been met (e.g., decreased thoughts about food). Additionally, considering how foods work together to produce satisfaction may help you and your client identify combinations of foods that will meet their nutritional needs.

For clients who cannot rely on fullness cues, setting minimums (in collaboration with a dietitian) may be necessary to ensure their nutritional needs are met.

Considerations for Group Interventions

In this session, you'll be discussing barriers to fullness and planning a paired snack activity. Unless you have a group with similar presenting concerns, each member is likely to encounter different barriers to fullness. Some members may associate feeling full with eating too much, and habitually stop short of feeling full. Other members may habitually eat in the absence of hunger and struggle to identify comfortable fullness. Because eating- and food-related matters are often coded as "good" or "bad" in our culture, what feels safe for one group member to discuss may not feel safe for others. To help make the group a safe space for everyone, emphasize that no barrier to fullness is "better" or "worse" than another—they're just different.

Planning for the between-session paired snack activity could also elicit comparisons among group members, as it may involve members sharing specific foods they will eat. If you judge that discussing specific foods will be triggering for members of your group, you can ask them to be more general when sharing their plans for the activity. For instance, group members might name food groups instead of specific foods (e.g., "This week I'll try adding protein to my afternoon snack") or share other details, like the days they plan to complete the activity.

You can also remind your group that context is key, and that while one person's snack may seem smaller or more nutritious, people's resources, needs, schedules, and preferences all vary.

Step 1: Between-Session Exercises Debriefing

Clients were asked to create a comprehensive inventory of the food-related beliefs they hold, critically evaluate these beliefs, and practice defusing from or reframing their unhelpful or inaccurate thoughts on the **Personal and Family Food Rules** handout. Check in with your client on the difficulty of this exercise. Were there any sticking points? For example, was it relatively easy to evaluate their beliefs, but harder to respond to them? Were they unsure which strategy they should use to respond to inaccurate or unhelpful thoughts? Did it feel mentally taxing to try to reframe their unhelpful thoughts?

When someone is attempting to change their thought patterns or behaviors, I like to use the analogy of learning to drive a car. Initially, every single step requires attention and intention. You have to think through putting on your seatbelt, adjusting the mirrors, checking your blind spot. With practice and time, however, much of the process becomes automatic. If you've been driving awhile, you're likely halfway down the road without any recollection of putting your seatbelt on. Similarly, the more your client practices cognitive defusion and reframing strategies, the more automatic they'll become. Early in the process, unhelpful thoughts will slip through and your client won't always have the bandwidth to reframe each one. This is normal! When cognitive reframing feels too emotionally taxing, I often recommend cognitive defusion: taking a step back and observing thoughts without pressure to change them. Generally, attending to self-care helps us feel less overwhelmed, have more resources, and even experience fewer negative thoughts in the first place.

Your client was also asked to continue practicing **Responding to Food- and Eating-Related Comments**. Check in on how it went. What comments came up during the week? What responses did they come up with, either in the moment or later? If there were any challenging comments or situations to navigate, brainstorm with your client how they might respond in the future.

Step 2: Overview of Feeling Your Fullness

Just as we sometimes have a fairly narrow view of what hunger feels like, it's common (and understandable) to think fullness is just feeling physically full. However, fullness comes with many other subtle signs. The following exercise is designed to help your client discover the subtle and not-so-subtle ways their body communicates fullness. Many factors can affect how in touch someone feels with their fullness cues. Some folks may be used to eating past comfortable fullness, and may struggle to identify it sooner. Others may associate fullness with eating too much, and may strive to stay shy of it. I've worked with people who really never feel full, either because these signals are inaccessible to them or because they don't eat enough to feel them. Since many people get disconnected from their fullness, start this work with your client by outlining the ways our bodies communicate that their needs have been met. This exercise should illuminate how accessible your client's fullness cues are and whether they experience any unique barriers to fullness, all of which will be useful in guiding future work. Bypass any questions that don't seem relevant to your client.

Session 5: Fullness and Satisfaction

EXERCISE: How Do I Know When I'm Full?

1. **When you think of fullness, what comes to mind?**

    Answers to this can vary widely. Your client might respond by talking about the *purpose* of fullness, or they may describe how fullness feels. Fullness may have a positive or negative valence for them, or it may be essentially neutral.

2. **What do you think the purpose of fullness is? Why do we feel it?**

    By this point in the intervention, your client has probably understood that our bodies send us signals for a reason. Still, because we're bombarded with messages about how much, when, and what to eat, the purpose of our hunger and fullness cues can get drowned out. So, ask this question if you feel your client could use reinforcement of this point.

3. **What do you notice when you feel full?**

    Your client might feel a general fullness or heaviness in their stomach, maybe accompanied by a sensation of bloating (which is normal). They will likely notice fewer thoughts about food. Food may become less exciting or may not taste quite as good. Eating will likely slow down. Their energy levels may rise or they may feel drowsy. If they were extremely hungry when beginning to eat, they might shift from being irritable to feeling like themselves again. They may become more relaxed and content.

4. **What do you notice is different when you feel comfortably full versus when you feel uncomfortably full?**

    Comfortable fullness is a subjective experience. However, typically it has a pleasant quality (usually 6 to 8 on the **Hunger Rating Scale**). Clients might feel content and like their needs were met. They could probably eat a few more bites, but not many more. Uncomfortable fullness is often a feeling of being "stuffed." One may feel nauseated, bloated, or tired, and experience regret or shame. Uncomfortable fullness can range from mildly unpleasant to very unpleasant (usually 9 to 10 on the **Hunger Rating Scale**). Often this level of fullness takes several hours to dissipate. However, remind clients who experience distress when they eat past satiety that inevitably fullness *does* decrease. Though it's unpleasant, even distressing, the feeling won't last forever. And, importantly, their bodies will need food again soon.

Almost everyone eats past comfortable fullness sometimes. In certain contexts (e.g., major holidays), eating past fullness is the norm! If a person knows it'll be a long time before they can eat again, eating past fullness may be the healthiest option—clients may work long shifts with few, if any, opportunities to eat. Eating more than they normally would before the shift may be important for them to have the necessary energy and mental resources. For people who are food insecure, eating past fullness may be a matter of survival.

This week, your client will complete the **Getting to Know Your Fullness** worksheet, which is especially helpful for those who feel disconnected from their hunger cues. Using the **Hunger Rating Scale**, your client will rate their *fullness* levels before and after two or three meals. They'll observe how long their fullness lasts by checking in every thirty minutes after the meal. This exercise is most useful when it's paired with meals they eat often. The goal is increased awareness of how they experience fullness. It can also provide insight into the staying power of meals they eat regularly (we'll explore this later in the session).

Step 3: Barriers to Feeling and Honoring Fullness

Once your client is acquainted with the why and how of fullness, it's time to consider what factors might get in the way of experiencing and honoring fullness cues.

EXERCISE: Exploring Barriers to Fullness

Brainstorm with your client or group potential things that may get in the way of their experiencing fullness. There are many possibilities; I list the most common barriers to fullness below, accompanied by brief descriptions. You can start this discussion by asking something like, "Many things can make it challenging to identify when we're full. Now that you've had a chance to think about how your body experiences fullness, what are some things you think get in the way?"

Common barriers to fullness your client identifies may include the following, which are further described below the list:

- Choosing foods that are not satisfying (fullness becomes harder to achieve)
- Fears of fullness
- Early satiety
- Eating quickly
- Eating when distracted
- Habitually eating the same amount regardless of hunger
- Inadequate self-care
- Low interoceptive awareness
- Mental health concerns
- Not eating until extreme hunger is reached
- Social pressures
- Struggling to identify comfortable fullness (potentially due to routinely eating to discomfort)
- Timing

Choosing Foods That Aren't Satisfying Satiety is contextual, and depends on amount consumed, type and combination of foods, hunger level before eating, emotions, energy, and more. Many diets promote eating combinations and amounts of foods that are unsatisfying. It's challenging (if not impossible) to feel full on many calorie-restricted diets. When calories are restricted, people often gravitate toward high-volume, low-density foods ("air foods"). If someone is eating rice cakes without adequate protein and fat, for instance, it's unlikely they will feel full (*or* satisfied). Some people may be limited in the types of foods available to them; take care to not villainize packaged or convenience foods. These can sometimes be less filling and satisfying, so it may take some brainstorming to figure out combinations of available foods that will aid satiety. The biggest priority is that your client is nourished.

Early Satiety Early satiety is not a barrier to identifying fullness so much as a barrier to adequate nourishment. If your client feels full soon after beginning to eat and there's no clear medical indication, referral to a physician is warranted. However, for clients with known conditions leading to early satiety (including recovery from an eating disorder), you may need to be savvy with food combinations. Consultation with a dietitian is extremely helpful when possible. Often, you want to look for low-volume, nutrient-dense foods you can pair or add. Fats are especially helpful for adding calories without adding much bulk; think adding peanut butter or coconut oil to a smoothie or oatmeal, putting avocado or butter on toast, choosing full-fat options like whole-milk yogurt and cottage cheese, and eating eggs *with* the yolk. As always, take into consideration your client's resources and the foods available to them.

Eating Quickly When we eat rapidly, we're less likely to sense emerging signs of fullness. It can take time for the body to catch up, which can lead to feeling uncomfortably full. For clients who eat rapidly, and often past comfortable fullness, it can help to work on slowing down eating. They could choose a few times over the next week when they have time to sit down for a meal. Ideally, they note their hunger level before the meal. Then, taking one bite at a time, they tune in to the eating experience, observing the tastes and textures of the food. I usually ask clients to pause about halfway through (sometimes it's even helpful to set a timer for five minutes) and check in with their fullness. They can ask themselves, does the food still taste as good? What am I noticing in my body? Is fullness emerging, or am I still hungry? The goal is *not* to eat less, but to begin familiarizing themselves with the early signs of satiety.

Eating When Distracted Distracted eating is common, and it's not always a problem. I've had many clients relay the experience of sitting down in front of the TV with a snack and soon realizing it's all gone. This can be disappointing, because they didn't get to really enjoy the food. In fact, when someone misses out on the pleasure of eating, they're more likely to go back for more, even when they're no longer physically hungry. Distracted eating means we're less tuned in to our bodies and thus less likely to notice emerging fullness.

Eating without distractions is simply not feasible for every meal or snack; I tell my clients that distracted eating is better than not eating. For instance, if a client has class all day and work in the evening, they may only have time to eat in the car. In that case, I'd rather my client distractedly eat than not eat at all. If distracted eating seems to be a barrier to fullness for your client, there are likely small ways to adjust, such as choosing to eat a couple of meals at the table without screens each week. See the **Distracted Eating** handout for more information.

Some people may *need* distraction to eat. I've worked with people with ARFID or in early eating disorder recovery who relied on distractions to get through meals. Again, the priority is that your client's needs are met. If distractions help your client nourish themselves adequately, then decreasing distracted eating may not be the right goal for them.

Fears of Fullness Some clients may find fullness aversive, even scary. This could be related to heightened sensitivity to gastrointestinal sensations, especially common in ARFID. Clients may have developed an association that fullness reflects *over*eating or feeling full may generate feelings of guilt or shame. Therefore, they may fear the sensation of fullness because it may evoke unbearable or distressing feelings (as in ARFID), or feelings that one has overeaten or done something wrong.

Unless exposure exercises are contraindicated, I recommend graduated exposures to help your client learn to tolerate feelings of *comfortable* fullness (understanding it likely won't feel comfortable initially). So, if your client always stops at one piece of pizza, you could try adding another half slice. If they're still experiencing signs of hunger, they could try two slices next time. But, as always, if they're hungry and willing to eat more in the moment, encourage that! Importantly, this activity should be paired with response prevention so your client doesn't engage in compensatory behaviors (which would negate the benefit of the exposures).

Habitually Eating the Same Amount Regardless of Hunger Many clients have told me they tend to eat whatever is on their plate, regardless of their hunger levels. Humans are creatures of habit; this isn't a bad thing! If everything we did required cognitive effort, we wouldn't get much done. However, habitually eating the same amount means we're relying on external cues (an amount on a plate) versus internal ones. Small adjustments might help—for instance, pausing to note hunger levels before plating the meal. If your client regularly plates more food than they're hungry for, they can practice putting less on their plate to start. However, it's vital that they understand they have *unconditional permission* to eat until satisfied. So, if the amount they add to their plate doesn't satisfy their hunger, they can get more.

Sometimes people are reluctant to leave or waste any food. Discuss some ways to repurpose leftovers, such as omelets, stir-fry, and rice or noodle bowls. Groups are especially great for brainstorming creative solutions to prevent food waste.

Inadequate Self-Care Deficits in self-care can disrupt interoceptive awareness. If your client has experienced a change in their ability to access their fullness cues, has begun eating past fullness more often, or is experiencing low appetite, assess for sleep, hydration, nutrition, stress, physical activity (is activity adequately nourished?), mental health, and food and housing security. Once self-care needs are addressed, interoceptive awareness *should* improve.

Low Interoceptive Awareness This can occur with medical conditions (or with their treatment), dieting or restriction, eating disorders, autism, ADHD, and exercise, which can carry increased nutritional needs. In these instances, fullness may not be a reliable barometer of adequate nutrition. As outlined in Session 2, clues that your client's nutritional needs are not being

Session 5: Fullness and Satisfaction   107

met include decreased energy, poor recovery (especially for athletes), poor sleep, brain fog, irritability, hormonal disruptions (e.g., irregular or missed periods), and getting sick more frequently. Your client may need to engage in mechanical eating and take note of other signs of satiation beyond the physical sensation of fullness (e.g., mood changes). If you're not a dietitian, collaborating with one is helpful here.

Mental Health Concerns Mental health concerns can disrupt interoceptive awareness. Self-care and mental health needs should be addressed first. If you're a mental health care provider and mental health concerns (e.g., depression) are precluding progress in intuitive eating, you may need to pause your work to focus on addressing your client's emotional needs. If you're not a mental health care provider, referrals to mental health resources will be important so your client has the capacity to focus on intuitive eating.

Not Eating Until Extreme Hunger Is Reached When a person doesn't eat until their hunger is extreme, whether voluntary or involuntary, they're more likely to eat rapidly and miss emerging signs of fullness. When one is food insecure, eating as much as possible when food is available is adaptive; addressing food insecurity should be the priority. For people who are food secure, assess for ways to increase the regularity of eating. For instance, meal prep is often challenging to prioritize but can be clutch during busy weeks. Sometimes, it's as simple as encouraging your client to always have snacks on hand.

Social Pressure Social pressure can lead people to eat past fullness. This pressure may be implicit, such as when others are eating more around you. It can also be explicit, such as family members encouraging you to clean your plate or get another helping. When social pressure is implicit, it's often a matter of being mindful and intentional. If your client notices they often eat past fullness when they're in a group, you could identify an upcoming social event where they can practice tuning in and being intentional (not distracted). It's trickier when someone is experiencing *explicit* pressure to eat past fullness. Your client can complete the **Clean Your Plate Club** handout for further reflection. You might consider doing a role-play with your client to practice communicating their needs and setting boundaries with loved ones.

Struggling to Identify Comfortable Fullness This may be due to routinely eating to discomfort. As with the recommendations given above for distracted, rapid, and habitual eating, your client may want to choose a few meals over the next week to practice slowing down eating, checking in with their fullness before eating, and setting a timer to check in midway through eating. These strategies should help them notice the subtle ways fullness emerges. Consult the **Stopping When Full** handout for more information.

Timing The spacing of meals affects fullness. Long stretches without eating can lead to primal hunger and, potentially, to binge episodes. Meals and snacks eaten close together can lead to early satiety. Meal timing won't always be modifiable; if your client needs to eat something because they won't have another opportunity to eat for many hours, they may have to eat when not very hungry. When meal timing isn't modifiable, your client may have to be more thoughtful about *what* they're eating. We'll get into this in the next section. Essentially, your client should consider choosing foods with staying power when they must go long stretches without eating and less filling foods when they'll need to eat again soon.

Optional Handouts

Your client may need or want more time exploring these barriers. There are optional handouts included with this chapter (**Distracted Eating, Clean Your Plate Club, Stopping When Full**) that you can assign for between-session reflection. Just take a little time in the next session to debrief.

The goal of the discussion about barriers to fullness is to identify which are modifiable. If you and your client identified modifiable barriers, make a goal to address one this week. In a group setting, members can brainstorm ideas together. Ideally, the goal will be something your client can practice a few times before the next session. For example, if your client engages in distracted eating that is *not* adaptive for them, perhaps identify three meals or snacks where they can sit at the table without any screens. Or, if your client grew up with a "clean your plate" mentality and now struggles to leave any food, even when no longer hungry, they might practice slowing down their eating and finding creative ways to repurpose leftovers. They can log their goal and progress on the **Barriers to Fullness** worksheet, which also has some questions for further reflection.

Step 4: Discovering the Staying Power of Foods

Many people aren't aware of how different foods affect fullness. When so many popular diets promote cutting out entire macronutrients, people may not realize that the macronutrients (protein, fat, carbohydrate) work together to influence satiety and satisfaction.

> ### Macronutrients 101
>
> **Carbohydrates** are the preferred energy source for many bodily tissues and the primary energy source for the brain. They help maintain normal blood sugar levels and aid muscle contractions during exercise. Fiber adds bulk and slows the absorption of carbohydrates into the bloodstream, thereby aiding fullness. Carbohydrates are found in simple forms (e.g., sugar) and complex forms (e.g., whole grains). Some foods have both (apples have sugar, a simple carb, and fiber, a complex carb). Simple carbs break down and enter the bloodstream more quickly, which is useful when quick energy is needed, while complex carbs break down more slowly, which can prolong fullness.
>
> **Fats** slow the digestion rate and prolong fullness. They also protect the organs and help the body absorb essential nutrients. They are found in nuts, oils, butter, full-fat dairy products, some meats and seafood (e.g., beef, salmon), and certain produce (e.g., avocados).
>
> **Protein** increases satiety and is involved in digestion (enzymes are proteins). It's crucial to the growth, development, repair, and maintenance of body tissue. It's found in animal sources (meat, seafood, dairy) and non-animal sources (beans, legumes, nuts, quinoa, soy).

Session 5: Fullness and Satisfaction   109

To the right is some basic nutrition information intended to illustrate how crucial each macronutrient is to our energy levels, satiety, and satisfaction. If you perceive your client isn't ready to talk about nutrition in this detail yet, you can simply communicate that carbohydrates, protein, and fat all perform essential functions that keep our bodies running.

EXERCISE: Snack Pairing Experiment

Diets often recommend foods without staying power, meaning fullness is fleeting and satisfaction is lacking. This can be frustrating, as your client might feel physically full but still desire food. Or they might feel hungry again quickly, which can be confusing. The following exercise helps generate awareness of how different food combinations impact satiety and satisfaction. This is ideal for those who sometimes feel unsatisfied after meals or snacks, find they are hungry again quickly, or frequently eat foods without staying power.

Before the next session, ask your client to pick a couple of days to experiment with how different snack pairings impact fullness and satiety. Ideally, they would choose a snack they eat regularly that they notice doesn't have staying power. Or you can use the **Snack Pairings** handout to generate ideas about combinations to try. For best results, your client would pick two days where they can hold the timing and content of their other meals and snacks constant. The handout has space to write the details of the goal, log progress, and reflect.

As an example, let's say your client works in the office on Mondays, Wednesdays, and Thursdays. These days are pretty routine: they eat the same or similar breakfast, lunch, and snack each day. They typically eat yogurt in the afternoon, but notice they're often ravenous when they get home, and they sometimes binge in the evening. To do this experiment, they could hold everything else constant on Monday and Wednesday, but vary their afternoon snack. On Monday they could eat their usual yogurt, log their fullness and satisfaction after, and then note how long it takes for their hunger to reemerge. On Wednesday, they could eat the yogurt alongside nuts and a piece of fruit, again logging their fullness and satisfaction levels when they finish eating and noticing how long they last.

Importantly, encourage your client to honor their hunger *as soon as it reemerges*. If they remain hungry after the snack, encourage them to eat more. You are absolutely not encouraging restriction here. The goal is to increase your client's awareness of how different food pairings may help increase the satisfaction and staying power of their meals and snacks. Additionally, you don't want to ask them to eat less than they normally would: if they usually have yogurt, almonds, and a banana for a snack, don't encourage them to just eat yogurt one day. Instead, is there another meal or snack your client has noticed lacks staying power? What could they add to round it out and increase satiety?

Step 5: Overview of the Satisfaction Factor

Eating is inherently pleasurable; it's not only necessary for survival, but is a primary way we form and maintain social connections. Yet, many people experience guilt about enjoying eating. I often use my dog as an example of how natural it is to enjoy food. My dog eats twice per day every single day; he's missed one meal in his entire life, which was the morning he had to fast for his dental cleaning. He knows and trusts food will be presented every day. Nevertheless, there is nothing, *nothing* more exciting to him than food. The moment I pull out one of his dental chews, he is overcome with joy and his tail wags the entire time he eats it. Although it may seem like a silly analogy, it's unlikely anyone is judging their pet for being excited about eating: it's just natural.

Satisfaction is *not* just about enjoyment. The sense of contentment experienced after a meal may signal that one's needs were met. For instance, you're unlikely to feel satisfaction and contentment after eating a bowl of lettuce, because lettuce is unlikely to meet your nutritional needs at any given time. If you add fat, protein, and carbohydrate sources to the lettuce, the chances are much greater you'll feel satisfied after eating until comfortable fullness. When a client mentions they don't feel satisfied after eating, I get curious about the typical composition of their meals. Often, a key macronutrient is missing.

Cravings are closely linked with satisfaction. People often feel guilty about cravings, seeing them as evidence of their emotional attachment to food. Yet, cravings *can* be a way the body communicates its nutritional needs. Cravings for chocolate could signal that someone needs more magnesium. Cravings for peanut butter may denote a need for fat and protein. We'll dive into emotional eating in the next session, but early in intuitive eating (if ever), I don't want clients overthinking their cravings.

But What Do I Want to Eat?

People are not always aware of *what* they want to eat. Some folks may get into thought spirals when choosing foods, ping-ponging between what *actually* sounds good and what they think they *should* eat. Others may be limited in the foods available to them. Some may experience periods of food insecurity, meaning what they *want* takes a necessary backseat to what is *available*. Others may habitually eat the same things, which may be necessary given the circumstances of their lives.

Not everyone will have the privilege to eat what they want when they want. And it's not realistic for anyone to do so all the time. However, if your client struggles to make decisions around food, the **Sensory Considerations** worksheet (adapted from *The Intuitive Eating Workbook*; Tribole & Resch, 2017) can help. It has questions to help your client identify what taste, texture, aroma, temperature, and appearance of food they're wanting. When piloting this intervention, my colleagues and I were surprised by how enthusiastically this worksheet was received. Group leaders mentioned saving it on their phones and using it as a reference when *they* felt unsure about what to eat. The worksheet includes reflection questions if your client routinely struggles to identify what foods sound good to them.

Step 6: Between-Session Exercises and Closing

This week, there are options for between-session exercises depending on the needs of your client. The **Getting to Know Your Fullness** exercise is designed to increase your client's awareness of how fullness feels in their body, with the help of the **Hunger Rating Scale**. If your client experiences barriers to fullness, they can complete the **Barriers to Fullness** exercise. The **Snack Pairings** exercise helps your client learn how different food combinations aid (or hinder) fullness. Finally, they can complete the **Sensory Considerations** worksheet or one of the optional exercises in Step 6. My recommendation is not to assign more than two exercises—you want your client to have practice but not be overwhelmed or oversaturated.

This is a jam-packed session, so I've focused on the fundamentals of fullness and satisfaction. Nevertheless, there may be additional topics your client needs more time on. Therefore, I have included a few additional resources and exercises, including an additional **Distracted Eating** activity, a handout about the **Clean Your Plate Club** (especially helpful if your client grew up in a house where they had to eat all their food), and an additional exercise for those who struggle with **Stopping When Full**. You can choose those most relevant for your client.

Closing

As always, make sure to close out the session by summarizing the discussion and asking your client what worked for them from the session.

Lengthening the Session

If time and resources permit, this session can be expanded into two. Lengthening this session may be useful if your client:

- Feels disconnected from their fullness cues or struggles to identify comfortable fullness
- Has a history of an eating disorder
- Has a history of food insecurity
- Experiences considerable barriers to self-care

To lengthen this session, I suggest:

- Spending the first session on Steps 2 and 3
- Spending the second session on Steps 4 and 5; if this session feels light, you can incorporate some optional activities

Shortening the Session

If clients have diminished interoceptive awareness, you may want to spend more time helping your client to identify less obvious signs of fullness, like fewer thoughts about food, and any barriers that could get in the way of fullness. Otherwise, you might want to focus on how your client can get their needs met in the absence of consistent fullness cues. This may involve discussion of the staying power of foods. It's important to at least briefly introduce what satisfaction is and why it's important to eating.

CHAPTER 9

Session 6: The Role of Emotions

Session Outline

Step 1: Between-Session Exercises Debriefing

    Getting to Know Your Fullness

    Barriers to Fullness

    Snack Pairings

    Optional: Sensory Considerations, Distracted Eating, Clean Your Plate Club, Stopping When Full

Step 2: Overview of the Role of Emotions in Eating

    Quick Q&A: How Do I Manage Stress?

Step 3: Checking Back In on Self-Care

    Quick Check-In: Was It Really My Emotions?

Step 4: Exploring the Role of Emotions in Eating and Exercise

    Exercise: Evaluating the Functions and Consequences of Emotional Eating

Step 5: Cultivating New Coping Strategies

    Exercise: Why Do We Have Emotions?

    Handout: Functions of Emotions

    Handout: Types of Coping

    Optional Handout: Urge Surfing

Step 6: Between-Session Exercises and Closing

    Emotional Eating Triggers

    Coping Log

    Types of Coping

Materials

Functions of Emotions

Types of Coping

Urge Surfing (optional)

Emotional Eating Triggers

Coping Log

Session Aim

Food and eating are intimately tied to our emotions. We bond with our caregivers through feeding, and connect over and celebrate with food. Food can be joyful and comforting. However, in a society in which many people go hungry, bodies are politicized, and contrasting messages about food and eating bombard us, eating can be fraught. It's no surprise that eating *isn't* always so joyful and that sometimes it becomes a tool to navigate challenging emotions.

Although we tend to think of turning *toward* food as "emotional eating,"[26] people use food or exercise to regulate emotions in many ways, including (but not limited to) bingeing, restriction, and compulsive exercise. Generally, these behaviors serve to help people gain a sense of comfort, or of safety, warmth, distraction, dissociation, control, elation, or achievement. We never want to fully remove the emotions from eating—it's likely not possible, and if it were, we'd be removing one of life's greatest pleasures. The problem arises when a person's *primary* way of regulating their emotions is through maladaptive eating or exercise behaviors. This session is designed to help your client explore the ways they may use eating or exercise to meet emotional needs. The goal is to expand your client's coping toolkit so that they have additional *constructive* ways to meet their emotional needs.

Additional Considerations and Potential Adaptations

This session provides an overarching view of the role emotions can play in eating and exercise. Rarely is it so simple as one emotion leading to one maladaptive behavior. A client may feel sad and turn to food to self-soothe, or feel overwhelmed and turn to restriction to numb. More likely, though, your client has developed complex associations among emotions, eating, and exercise in response to layered challenges. For instance, some people (especially those in marginalized bodies) may wish to shrink themselves to feel safe in an unsafe world. Others may attempt to change their body because their sex at birth doesn't align with their gender. This session will give your client a chance to explore how emotions interact with their eating and exercise and to consider additional coping strategies they can incorporate. You may need to make space to process the injustices and challenges your client faces that they *can't* single-handedly change, and have empathy for the ways they've attempted to take care of themselves through these experiences. The outcome of this session should not be that your client feels the very real hardships and barriers they experience are minimized, nor should they get the sense that their provider thinks a changed mindset or new coping strategy will solve all their problems. Rather, we're attempting to alleviate suffering and increase your client's quality of life.

---

26   I'll use "emotional eating" throughout this session as shorthand. Please be aware that "emotional eating" is not confined to eating to cope with emotions, but can also look like restriction or maladaptive exercise behaviors.

Session 6: The Role of Emotions

> ## Considerations for Group Interventions
>
> If your group is heterogenous in terms of eating concerns, be mindful of how you present the information in this session. Emphasize throughout that "emotional eating" looks different for everyone (and can vary for each individual, too). Further, because restriction and excessive exercise are often equated with willpower and strength, whereas bingeing or emotional eating are often equated with a *lack* of willpower, some members may feel more comfortable speaking up in this session than others. It can bear repeating to participants that we don't see *any* form of maladaptive eating or exercise as better than another. Restriction and exercise can be as damaging as eating past fullness or bingeing, if not more so.
>
> In Step 4, your group will explore the functions and consequences of "emotional eating." The goal of this exercise is to identify the functions of these behaviors in order to generate empathy and insight. When piloting this intervention, my colleagues and I did not adequately convey the exercise's purpose and were dismayed when group members began to cite the benefits of maladaptive behaviors (e.g., saving money when restricting food) and not these behaviors' functions. Be mindful of how you present the purpose of this exercise. Your group may also identify several functions these behaviors serve, which could result in a longer list of functions than consequences. It's not about the length of the lists, but the relative weight of each item. There may be many ways maladaptive eating and exercise behaviors function to meet emotional needs, but they likely come at considerable cost.

Step 1: Between-Session Exercises Debriefing

Because the last session had a lot of content to cover, exercise options were provided. Your client may have completed the **Getting to Know Your Fullness, Barriers to Fullness, Snack Pairings,** and/or **Sensory Considerations** exercises. There were also optional exercises you may have assigned, including **Distracted Eating, Clean Your Plate Club,** and **Stopping When Full.**

Getting to Know Your Fullness Explore the patterns your client observed. How able were they to identify their fullness? Was it a challenge to note emerging or comfortable fullness? What did they notice about *how* their body communicated fullness? Did certain meals stick with them longer than others? Hopefully they're noticing that snacks and meals with adequate portions of ALL macronutrients are the most satisfying. Fat and protein add satisfaction and staying power, and carbs are important for energy. Eating foods with staying power will likely help your client feel better physically and have more energy to get through their day. It's important to remind clients in the context of this principle that intuitive eating is *not* the hunger/fullness diet. Some days, the best choice may be for them to eat past comfortable fullness if they won't be able to eat again for a while. They may sometimes eat past fullness in social situations or at celebrations, or because they went too long without eating. All of that is normal!

Barriers to Fullness Check in with your client on their exploration of decreasing a barrier to fullness they experience. If it went well, they could try next week to practice decreasing a different barrier (or stay the course). Troubleshoot if they couldn't address the barrier: maybe it isn't actually a problem, maybe it's not modifiable, or maybe adjustments are needed.

Snack Pairings Check in on which snacks they tried. How much were they able to hold other variables constant (e.g., meal content or timing)? What did they notice about the different combinations? Which snack had more staying power? Also check that they honored their hunger (if possible) when it emerged. Hopefully, they realize that when they choose foods with more staying power, they not only feel better physically but no longer have so many distracting thoughts about food.

Sensory Considerations This exercise was hopefully a fun one! Did your client learn anything about their preferences over the week? Did any patterns emerge? For instance, I notice that my body naturally adapts; when I have eaten a sweeter meal, I often (but not always) gravitate toward a savory option later in the day. Additionally, I've learned that I almost always crave contrasting textures. I like crunchy peanut butter, dark chocolate with sea salt and almonds, and so on. My preferences aren't any better than those of someone who prefers smooth peanut butter or milk chocolate—they're just different. Understanding my preferences better helps me reduce *some* indecision around choosing foods.

Step 2: Overview of the Role of Emotions in Eating

There are many ways we use food or exercise to cope with or navigate challenging emotions. Doing so looks different for everyone, and it may look different for your client from day to day. For instance, it's common to turn to food for comfort when sad or as a distraction when bored, and to lose your appetite when anxious. Emotions also affect our body image. Research shows that body image fluctuates in response to a variety of factors, including social interactions, negative affect, exercise, and mood (Fuller-Tyszkiewicz, 2019). Modern life is increasingly stressful, and the twenty-four-hour news cycle and ubiquity of social media can make it hard to find respite. Even for someone with a wide repertoire of effective coping skills and privileges, it can be hard to cope with life's many demands and stressors. Many people face disproportionate stress and hardship; others were not shown effective ways to cope with challenges and difficult emotions. The point is: if your client struggles with some form of emotional eating, we want to normalize and decrease the shame around that. At some point, coping with emotions through food or exercise may have been the only way they could meet their needs. The goal now is to gain awareness of any emotional eating patterns and determine whether these patterns are ultimately serving your client's goals and values.

Introduce the above considerations before jumping into the following questions. The questions in the quick Q and A below are general, because emotional eating looks so different depending on the person and context. Modify to make them specific for your client. The goal is to begin generating insight before diving deeper into the functions of emotional eating later in the session.

Session 6: The Role of Emotions

QUICK Q&A: How Do I Manage Stress?

1. **How do you typically manage your stress?**

2. **What ways do you think you may use food or exercise to cope?**

    Any behavior, whether it's restriction, eating past fullness, or exercise can be a coping strategy.

3. **Do you have ideas about how these patterns developed?**

    The goal is to generate insight and decrease any shame your client may have by providing context about how these patterns developed. If coping with emotions via food or exercise was modeled by family, the goal is not to place blame. Families do the best they can with the tools they have.

Step 3: Checking Back In on Self-Care

For clients who perceive they eat in response to emotions, consider whether they're *actually* eating emotionally. In Session 2, you covered the connection between self-care and interoceptive awareness. Deficits in self-care often have cascading consequences. For instance, when sleep is inadequate, we're not only likely to feel fatigued, but also potentially anxious, foggy, or irritable. Or, we may eat more to get that needed boost. Further, if your client still has a lingering diet mentality, they may eat in ways that feel out-of-control or emotional but are actually due to restriction (whether actual or mental).

In a group setting, validate that this content may not resonate with everyone. Nevertheless, if you have members who *do* perceive they emotionally eat, this material is important to cover. Below is a quick check-in to help your client identify whether their identified "emotional eating" is actually emotional.

QUICK CHECK-IN: Was It Really My Emotions?

Ask your client to imagine a time they perceived they ate a large amount of food or otherwise ate emotionally. Get curious with the following questions:

Were there new or additional stressors in their lives?

Had they been eating balanced, regular meals?

Had their activity levels changed?

Were they experiencing any physical changes (e.g., hormonal shifts, illness)?

Did their schedule shift such that they were eating at different times?

How were they sleeping?

Were they engaging in any mental or actual restriction?

It's possible these "emotional eating" episodes were actually due to biological hunger or a self-care deficit. If your client is satisfying their hunger but struggling with stress management or self-care, the remainder of the session will help you identify adaptive ways they can address their emotional needs. Self-care should always be addressed first, as it's the foundation upon which everything else rests.

Step 4: Exploring the Role of Emotions in Eating and Exercise

People cope with positive *and* negative emotions through eating and exercise. It's simply human to connect over and celebrate with food. We would never want to remove that source of joy and connection from life. Therefore, the purpose of the following exercise is to help your client delineate which forms of "emotional eating" bring them more harm than benefit or are otherwise not aligned with their values. This exercise should be guided with compassion, empathy, and curiosity, as maladaptive eating and exercise behaviors are functional, arising to meet real emotional needs.

EXERCISE: Evaluating the Functions and Consequences of Emotional Eating

This exercise works especially well when you make a visual. Ask your client to jot down a few recent times when they felt they used eating or exercise behaviors to cope.

While they're writing, create two columns with headings "Functions" and "Consequences." You'll note whether each function and consequence has short- or long-term effects, so leave room to write that in.

1. **Eating and exercise behaviors can be used to cope with a variety of emotions. What are some emotions that might be coped with this way?**

    Emphasize that these emotions can be positive or not. Common responses include being bored, stressed, tired, sad, lonely, happy, needing comfort, seeking celebration or connection, or feeling out of control, insecure, or anxious.

2. **What are some ways that coping through food or exercise has felt helpful to you in the past?**

    Write responses in the "Functions" column. For instance, clients may have experienced numbing, brief pleasure, distraction, comfort, or short-term anxiety relief. Importantly, some clients may cite what they perceive as *benefits* of these behaviors, which is distinct from how they *function* to meet emotional needs. For

Session 6: The Role of Emotions

instance, clients may save money when they restrict their food. Limited financial resources generate considerable stress. and one might argue that saving money through restriction alleviates such stress. However, short-term anxiety relief, *not* saving money, may be the function of restricting, so exploring the costs of these behaviors will be important.

3. **Now that we've identified some functions of these behaviors, let's consider how long the effects last.**

    For each function, identify whether the effects are short-term or long-term. Often, emotional eating behaviors have short-term effects because they're not addressing the root issues. For instance, if clients eat to soothe loneliness or sadness, how long does the soothing effect last? Or, if someone compulsively exercises to alleviate anxiety, how long do the anxiolytic effects last? They may discover that these effects are soon overtaken by rebound emotions, like shame.

4. **Let's talk about some of the consequences of these behaviors.[27] Let's approach this with nonjudgmental curiosity, knowing you've done the best you could at the time with the tools that were available.**

    Clients who eat in response to emotions may have an easier time identifying consequences because these behaviors are so harshly judged in many cultural contexts. Conversely, because the dominant culture celebrates restriction and extreme exercise, clients might have a harder time identifying the consequences of those behaviors. Give them time to think, but if they're struggling, offer a few ideas, such as isolation, physical discomfort, fatigue, weakness, or the numbing of positive feelings.

5. **How long do these consequences tend to last?**

    The consequences of such behaviors generally endure until the behaviors cease, and can compound over time. For instance, compulsive exercise may lead to injuries and illness, which will worsen if a person persists despite them. Similarly, social isolation could have compounding effects, as relationships may fracture or end.

6. **When looking at these lists, what do you notice?**

    Encourage them to compare not just the *length* of the lists, but also the weight of each item. The effects of these behaviors were likely temporary: bandages that didn't improve the underlying situation or discomfort. The consequences likely cost much more in the long run.

    Hopefully, by the end of this exercise your client will have increased insight about the functions and consequences of their maladaptive eating and exercise behaviors. This insight should facilitate continued reflection throughout the week, which you can fortify by providing the **Emotional Eating Triggers** handout to complete between sessions.

---

[27] Rather than framing this discussion around consequences, it may be more applicable or feel more salient to say, "In what ways are these behaviors out of alignment with your values?"

Step 5: Cultivating New Coping Strategies

Identifying the functions of maladaptive eating and exercise behaviors is a crucial first step to elucidating your client's underlying emotional needs. Emotions provide essential information about our needs.[28] When we don't recognize that emotions are functional, we might see them as a nuisance, become overly identified with them, or choose coping strategies that aren't well matched for the underlying need. For instance, your client may eat to self-soothe because they're distressed or sad. However, if they don't explore the underlying emotion, they may miss that the sadness or distress is related to feelings of loneliness or isolation. Although eating can be quite soothing in the short term, it's unlikely to provide someone with an enduring sense of support or connection. Exploring what function emotional eating is serving can help clients choose a more effective coping strategy.

I cannot stress this enough: it's *normal* and potentially even *adaptive* to cope through food or exercise sometimes. Movement can be a wonderful coping strategy provided it is not punishing, compulsive, or done despite injury or illness. If we had a bad day at work, buying a cookie and eating it on the way home could provide needed joy. The goal is that your client makes *intentional* decisions about how to cope and that they have tools available to them beyond restriction, eating, and exercise.

Use the **Functions of Emotions** and **Types of Coping** handouts to guide the following exercises. The **Functions of Emotions** handout details the overarching and specific functions of emotions. The **Types of Coping** handout references the types of coping strategies and when each type is likely to be most effective. For instance, distraction may be useful for nonproductive anxiety, whereas emotion-focused coping strategies like self-soothing may be helpful when dealing with disappointment. The goal of this exercise is to help clients identify their emotion, determine what that emotion is telling them about their needs or values, and identify an appropriate coping strategy.

EXERCISE: Why Do We Have Emotions?

1. **Why do you think humans have emotions? What purpose do they serve?**

   In the framework of dialectical behavior therapy (DBT; Linehan, 1993), emotions have three overarching functions. **(1) To motivate and organize us for action.** When we don't have time to think through a situation, emotions propel our action. Fear communicates that we need to fight, flee, or freeze. Anxiety can tell us that we need to plan and prepare for something in the future. Sadness can prompt us to seek social connection. **(2) To communicate with others.** Emotions can alert others to our needs. When a child cries, their caregiver perceives the child is distressed and is motivated to act. **(3) To communicate to ourselves.** Though they are sometimes bothersome or inconvenient, emotions let us know what we need. Feeling

---

[28] This section is guided by the work of psychologist Susan David, PhD. I highly recommend her book *Emotional Agility* for further reading.

Session 6: The Role of Emotions

disconnected from a partner can tell us there's something to address within our relationship.

2. **What about specific emotions? What might they tell us?**

   Fear tells us we perceive an immediate threat to our safety. Guilt tells us we've acted out of alignment with our values. Sadness may mean we're disappointed or it might communicate an underlying fear. Love means we feel connected and supported. The **Functions of Emotions** serves as a guide.

3. **Think of a recent time you used eating or exercise to cope with an emotion. What emotion do you think you were experiencing?**[29]

   Maybe your client felt rejected by a friend and turned to food to feel comforted. Or the behavior served a deeper function; for instance, if a client felt threatened in their environment due to their body size, race, gender, or sexuality, they might cope through food or exercise to make themselves smaller or larger. The handout has a list of emotions in case your client struggles to think of examples.

4. **Earlier, we talked about how eating and exercise behaviors can be quite effective in the short term. However, these effects rarely last and often have long-term consequences. Look at the** Types of Coping **handout and consider: What other ways might you cope if you feel that emotion come up again?**

   If, for example, your client felt rejected by a friend, they may have needed to engage in a self-soothing or distracting activity (emotion-focused coping), or they may have been ready to have a conversation with their friend (problem-focused coping). If your client is experiencing systemic discrimination that no amount of coping at the individual level is going to solve, it may be more helpful to consider if there are other ways they can take care of themselves or feel a sense of safety that cause them less harm. For instance, are there ways they can increase their sense of community connectedness and belonging? Are there different healthcare providers they can see? Do they need a referral to a trauma-focused therapist?

   Clients may sometimes be unable to identify their emotional needs because their feelings or urges are so intense, or because they're feeling overwhelmed and maxed out. When this happens, a technique called **Urge Surfing** can be especially helpful. Urge surfing is used across various psychotherapies (e.g., DBT, ACT, CBT) and in substance use disorder treatment. It likens heightened emotions and urges to waves that gradually build in intensity and peak before fading away. Thus, any strong emotion or urge your client is experiencing will diminish with time, and often, it's not long. To "surf" the wave, they use mindfulness. Rather than being reactive to their emotions, they sit with them. Since uncomfortable emotions are part of being human, it's important to develop the tools to sit with and *move through* them. Provide your client with the **Urge Surfing** handout to reference when needed.

---

29 Note that alexithymia (difficulty in identifying and describing experienced emotions) is common within eating disorders and among autistic individuals.

If clients feel the urge to deny themselves food, urge surfing helps them check in with their body's needs. Nourishment should help them think more clearly, which might help them identify how to cope with difficult emotions contributing to the urge to restrict. Similarly, if your client is experiencing an urge to eat and they're unsure whether it's emotional or biological hunger, pausing gives them the opportunity to check in with their body. If after pausing they're still unsure, I'd rather they eat! I prefer my clients *not* overthink hunger. If they eat and realize they weren't experiencing biological hunger, it's no big deal. They have great data for the future and any physical discomfort should dissipate relatively quickly.

Step 6: Between-Session Exercises and Closing

Between sessions, your client will use the **Emotional Eating Triggers** handout to identify and reflect on any situations or emotions that can trigger them to use restriction, eating, or exercise to cope. Additionally, clients can practice cultivating new coping strategies using the **Coping Log** to note when they experience a strong emotion. Instead of using a maladaptive eating or exercise behavior, they'll practice using one of the strategies discussed in session or listed on the **Types of Coping** handout. For instance, they may choose to use a problem- or emotion-focused coping strategy or engage in urge surfing when experiencing intense emotions or emotional eating urges. Ideally, they'll practice using an alternate coping strategy at least three times between sessions.

Closing

As always, close out the session with something that resonated with you both.

Lengthening the Session

If time and resources permit, this session can be expanded into two. Almost everyone could benefit from deeper emotional processing and more coping practice. However, it may be especially helpful to lengthen this session for clients who:

- Experience considerable emotional dysregulation
- Have co-occurring mental health diagnoses
- Experience disproportionate stigma or discrimination
- Are currently experiencing multiple or serious stressors (such as grief)

To lengthen this session, I suggest:

- Spending the first session on Steps 2 and 3
- Spending the second session on Steps 4 and 5

Shortening the Session

Alexithymia is common among autistic people. Collaborate with autistic clients on how much time would be useful to spend on the content related to emotional awareness; an autistic client's emotions (e.g., irritability) can be useful data that signal when they may need to eat. Be careful not to pathologize coping strategies that are adaptive for autistic clients. For clients with trauma histories, you can discuss the role of emotions in eating and exercise and the functions of emotions generally but may want to avoid deeper processing if you do not have trauma training. You may need to refer to a trauma specialist to avoid retraumatizing or causing more harm.

CHAPTER 10

Session 7: Body Respect

Session Outline

Step 1: Between-Session Exercises Debriefing
    Emotional Eating Triggers
    Coping Log

Step 2: Overview of Body Respect
    Body Diversity and Weight Science
    Other Body Image Concerns
    Exercise: Body Image Reflection

Step 3: Life Without Body Negativity
    Exercise: Imagining a Life with Body Respect

Step 4: Cultivating Body Respect
    Handout: Cultivating Body Respect
    The Harms of Self-Monitoring
    The Doctor's Office
    Handout: Tips for Navigating Doctor Visits
    Opposite Action: Treating the Body with Kindness

Step 5: Responding to Body Talk
    Exercise: Part 1—Options for Responding to Body Talk
    Exercise: Part 2—Role-Play of Body Talk Responses

Step 6: Social Media
    Handout: Social Media Strategies

Step 7: Between-Session Exercises and Closing
    Expand Your Horizon (Exercise #1)
    Negative Body Talk

Materials

Cultivating Body Respect

Tips for Navigating Doctor Visits

Social Media Strategies

Expand Your Horizon

Negative Body Talk

Session Aim

When most of us think of body image, we think of it as our perception of our appearance, shape, or size. From an early age many of us are imprinted with the notion that our physical appearance is integral to our worth and value as people. Because cultural parameters of a "good" appearance are extremely narrow, often unattainable, and ever evolving, striving to achieve these ideals is fruitless for most.

However, body image is much more complex than our perception of our physical appearance. Body image also encompasses our experience of living *in* our body (Piran, 2016). The concept of embodiment acknowledges that body image also includes internal experiences (attunement), experience of the body in relation to others, and the body's interactions with social structures such as stigma and oppression.

Drawing from the related concepts of body functionality appreciation, body neutrality, and fat liberation, body respect is, at its core, about learning to treat one's body with kindness, regardless of how it looks and functions. Through this work, you'll help your client develop appreciation for the functions of their body (Alleva et al., 2015). Recognizing that feeling *positively* about how one looks can be extremely challenging in our cultural milieu, you can help your client de-invest in the importance of appearance and embrace a neutral stance toward how they look. Through this work, your client's appearance (and how well it aligns with current societal ideals) will ideally no longer be a primary way they measure their self-worth. In the best-case scenario, your client will develop confidence to take up space in this world, inhabiting their body fully and without shame. Accepting and taking care of our body without trying to shrink it for others' comfort is a radical act. If your client doesn't get there, it's not a failure on their part but a reflection of a world that's unsafe for them to inhabit authentically. Therefore, the goals of this session are to help your client relate to their body in new ways and begin working toward honoring their body's needs. Because social media is a potent influence on people's body image, we'll touch on how to fortify your client against the threats social media pose to body esteem.

Additional Considerations and Potential Adaptations

We have abundant evidence that body image concerns are universal. Each person's culture, race, ethnicity, gender, sexual orientation, ability, size, shape, socioeconomic status, and age all intersect to affect how each of us feels about and *in* our bodies. Yet, historically, body image concerns have been viewed as superficial issues primarily affecting young, white women. The possibility of such concerns among men and other groups (e.g., Black women) has been ignored. This narrow perception has not only distorted research findings, but contributed to levels of stigma and bias that keep many from effective treatment. When doing body respect work with clients, it's important to stay mindful of your own biases and to consider how stigma could affect both your client's awareness of their body image concerns and their willingness to discuss those concerns. For instance, men may be less likely to recognize their own concerns as problematic and less likely to seek help due to stigma (Räisänen & Hunt, 2014).

As always, tailor your presentation of the information in this session to your client's unique concerns, including their identities. Body image pressures tend to differ across groups. Men experience greater pressure to obtain a lean, muscular physique, for instance, and appearance-related pressures appear heightened for gay men (Convertino et al., 2021; Lavender et al., 2017). Black women experience pressures to conform to both white appearance ideals (e.g., thinness) and those of their own cultural group (Capodilupo & Kim, 2014). Don't assume your client simply desires to be thinner, as their relationship with their body is likely more complex. Similarly, it's critical that information in this session, particularly around body functionality appreciation, is not presented in an ableist way. Body respect is possible regardless of ability status, but there are additional barriers for someone with a disability, or a chronic illness. It will likely be helpful to acknowledge that, rather than avoid it.

The goal of body respect is to reduce attempts at body modification that *increase* suffering and *reduce* quality of life. Gender-diverse clients may wish to modify their bodies to bring them in alignment with their gender identity, and research supports that gender-affirming interventions benefit quality-of-life and mental health overall (Almazan & Keuroghlian, 2021; Tordoff et al., 2022). So, for example, you will want to help your client decrease their use of maladaptive eating and exercise behaviors (those that hamper quality of life), while supporting them in pursuing gender-affirming interventions that can increase quality of life. Take care when introducing the idea of accepting one's genetic blueprint (covered in this chapter) with gender-diverse clients.

Considerations for Group Interventions

Group members will likely have differing body image concerns and experiences. Navigating group dynamics around these topics can be tricky! As always, be mindful of power differentials and comparisons among those in more socially accepted bodies and those in less socially accepted bodies, which may affect the ways various group members show up and speak up. Social comparisons are likely, and group members I've worked with have mentioned it was helpful to hear that being thin or conventionally attractive doesn't solve body image concerns. It may also be challenging for some group members to hear someone in a thin or conventionally attractive body discussing their body dissatisfaction. I like to name that people in the group will have differing experiences related to their appearance and identities, and acknowledge that some folks will experience more discrimination based on how they look.

Step 1: Between-Session Exercises Debriefing

Your client was asked to identify and reflect on **Emotional Eating Triggers**: situations and emotions that trigger their maladaptive eating and exercise. Did they notice any patterns? As always, approach this conversation with compassion. Their coping strategies likely served them in the past and were effective in the short term. The goal of this exercise was to generate insight about situations and emotions particularly likely to increase urges to use eating or exercise behaviors to cope. Hopefully, this insight facilitates greater mindfulness so your client can notice their emotions and choose a coping strategy with intention instead of being on autopilot. Ideally, your client begins to develop new coping strategies that are aligned with their values and provide more long-term benefit.

Your client was asked to complete a **Coping Log** where they noted urges to use maladaptive eating or exercise behaviors to manage difficult emotions. They were encouraged to consider other, more adaptive coping strategies when possible, such as urge surfing, self-soothing, or distracting. If they were experiencing biological hunger concurrent with a strong emotion or urge, they were encouraged to nourish themselves.

If your client was able to identify strong emotions or urges, acknowledge that as progress. Awareness is a crucial first step. If your client engaged in a maladaptive eating or exercise behavior in response to the emotion or urge, take a little time to explore what made choosing a different coping strategy challenging.

Clients may be initially disappointed when new coping strategies are not as immediately powerful as eating, compensatory behaviors, or restriction. Effective coping involves an amalgamation of different strategies, such as sleep, nutrition, mindfulness, distress tolerance, and social support, that fit together to promote quality of life. Combining these strategies should provide long-term benefit for clients, but you can hold space for the reality that they might not always be as potent in the short term. And we don't want to remove emotion from eating and exercise—especially not joy, pleasure, and connection. Rather, we want to add other strategies to your client's toolbox so that food and exercise behaviors are no longer the primary ones they reach for.

Step 2: Overview of Body Respect

The core components of body respect are accepting one's natural body size and developing an appreciation for one's body that extends beyond its appearance. This acceptance and appreciation should foster a more compassionate stance toward one's body, making it easier to honor bodily needs—and body appreciation is strongly linked to greater intuitive eating. However, generating acceptance and embracing body diversity can be challenging for many reasons. As you introduce this session, explore the unique barriers your client encounters to body respect. What could get in the way of them accepting their body and treating it with kindness?

Body Diversity and Weight Science

Many clients will have internalized the idea that thinner or fitter bodies are *healthier*. They may feel their efforts to change their bodies are genuinely in the interest of their health and longevity. Thus, although you will have touched on body diversity and weight science in the first session, it's helpful to revisit these concepts now.

Although bodies are naturally diverse and come in many shapes and sizes, we're led to believe that certain bodies are better than others, and we're encouraged to try to fit our bodies into narrow standards. Though we understand we cannot change our height, many of us work hard to change the appearance, shape, or size of other aspects of our bodies. And though some changes may be possible, especially in the short term, they often require enormous resources to attain and maintain. Our bodies are biologically primed to defend their set-point range (the weight at which they perform best) with numerous mechanisms to resist weight loss and starvation (Hall & Guo, 2017). Our bodies are smart! When we restrict, we have increased attentional biases toward food cues and are more likely to notice food in our environment (Stice et al., 2013). Foods become more rewarding, especially energy-dense ones. (Perhaps one reason why vegetables aren't quite as rewarding as other foods is that they take a lot of work for your body to digest with very little energy payoff;[30] Stice, Burger & Yokum, 2013.) As a person loses weight, they become more metabolically efficient—the body gets better at subsisting on less (MacLean et al., 2004). Indeed, there is evidence that metabolic adaptations can persist long after weight loss (Fothergill et al., 2016); these adaptations help the body survive the next famine. Yet, repeated attempts at weight loss are harmful, both psychologically and physically (Tomiyama, 2014). Hinging one's body esteem on a particular weight or shape can require near-constant micromanagement. Our bodies are meant to change throughout our lives.

Other Body Image Concerns

Many clients will have body image concerns that are not centered on the desire for weight loss or the belief that thinner is healthier. Some may feel that achieving a certain appearance is important for other reasons, such as acceptance from others, being desirable to potential dating partners, or feeling safe in a world that discriminates against them. Disabilities and illness can also profoundly affect a person's relationship with their body. People often experience deep grief or resentment over body-related changes resulting from cancer and its treatment, for instance.

Regardless of the nature of your client's body image concerns, it's valuable to help them consider whether feeling negatively toward or trying to change their body is worthwhile, especially when there's evidence intuitive eating can benefit one's physical and mental health (Linardon et al., 2021; Quansah et al., 2019). Encourage your client to reflect on what it might be like to begin to accept their body as it is.

EXERCISE: Body Image Reflection

These questions will help clients explore their relationship with their body. Not all will be relevant, so focus on those that are most pertinent.

1. **What is your relationship with your body currently like?**

    In a group setting, you may want to ask each person to spend a few moments privately reflecting on this question rather than sharing as a group.

2. **How important do you feel your appearance is to your sense of self-worth? What feels important about looking a certain way?**

---

30 Vegetables have *many* nutritional benefits and are loaded with key micronutrients, but they're *not* an efficient energy source.

Session 7: Body Respect

This question is most appropriate for clients invested in the importance of their appearance. For instance, if you have a male-identifying client who is preoccupied with gaining muscle or looking toned, explore what feels important about those appearance goals.

3. **What comes up when you think about embracing your body as it is? Do you have any fears?**

4. **Think of your closest friend, your partner, or a beloved family member. What do you love most about them? What characteristics make them a good, valuable person?**

    Most likely, appearance is at most a small part of why your client values their loved one. If they don't view their loved one's appearance as integral to their worth, why doesn't the same apply to themselves?

5. **If this loved one was struggling with their body image, what would you want for them?**

    Again, it's unlikely your client would want their loved one to feel negatively toward their body or spend valuable time and resources on changing it. What would it be like to see themselves as their loved ones do? What might that take?

Step 3: Life Without Body Negativity

Rodin, Silberstein, and Striegel-Moore (1985) coined the term *normative discontent* to describe the pervasive phenomenon of body dissatisfaction among women. Feeling bad about one's body is the rule, not the exception, and this phenomenon cuts across identity lines. Because body negativity is so normative, people don't often reflect on its consequences. The following exercise is intended to help your client consider the costs of body negativity for them. As you discuss it together, you can add nuance or context. If your client believes their body negativity is warranted because they *need* to change their body for health reasons, you can hold space for that belief. And you can explore with them what consequences in their life body negativity has created. If your client doesn't feel negatively about their body, you might instead frame the conversation around the consequences of devoting resources such as time, energy, and money toward changing their body.

EXERCISE: Imagining a Life with Body Respect

I recommend that you write out your client's responses to these questions on a whiteboard or a pad of paper. It's powerful to see a representation of life *with* body respect next to a representation of life *without* it.

1. **Imagine a life in the future where you feel at peace with and at home in your body. Your body is a place you feel comfortable inhabiting. You take care of your body like it belongs to someone you love. How your body looks is no longer a primary measure of your self-worth. You don't spend your valuable resources trying to change your body to fit others' expectations. What might you gain?**

    Write the ideas your client names on the left side of the paper or whiteboard. Some possibilities might be: more confidence to meet people and gain new connections; more concentration; likelier to meet education and career goals; freedom to choose movement or exercise that is enjoyable (not obligatory); freedom to enjoy meals out with loved ones; more time for hobbies and interests because less time is spent trying to modify appearance; money saved.

2. **Now, imagine a future where you don't accept your body. You dedicate your time and resources to changing it. What does this future look like? What might be the consequences?**

    Write the consequences your client mentions on the right side of the paper or whiteboard. Some possibilities might be: less time with loved ones; less confidence to meet new people or date (if interested); less concentration for school or work; less confidence to pursue social, school, or work opportunities; more time taken to change or modify appearance; less time for hobbies or other interests; money spent to change appearance; missing out on social occasions around food OR not enjoying social occasions around food.

3. **Let's compare these two futures. Which is more appealing? Which feels potentially more realistic? If you're interested in accepting your body or letting go of the struggle to change it, what would need to change for you to do so?**

    Validate your client for identifying ways their life might improve from letting go of body negativity or body modification, but also acknowledge the realistic difficulty of actually doing so! In the next step, you'll move from the *why* to the *how* by discussing habits your client can cultivate to work toward body respect.

Step 4: Cultivating Body Respect

Your client may not feel ready to accept their body's genetic blueprint. That's OK! Embrace that dialectic. Again, it can be unsafe to exist in a body that society has deemed problematic. Your client doesn't have to accept their body to begin making small steps toward body respect.

The first **Cultivating Body Respect** exercise is aimed at body functionality appreciation. If your client has been unhappy with their body for a long time, feeling grateful for it may seem unreachable. Yet, gratitude actually changes one's brain (Kini et al., 2016): the more you practice, the more automatic gratitude becomes. In fact, when you regularly practice gratitude, you start to *look for* things for which you're grateful.

Gratitude is not all-or-nothing. I have worked with people with cancer who feel betrayed by their body and no longer feel at home in a body changed by cancer and its treatment. Despite

Session 7: Body Respect

their many reasons for body negativity, they still benefit from fostering body appreciation. For instance, their body is working incredibly hard to fight the cancer and to heal from treatment! Thus, this exercise isn't intended to dismiss anyone's struggle, but to expand your client's view of their body and to help them relate to it in a new way. Their feelings toward their body are completely valid, and this exercise will not erase the circumstances that make body appreciation so hard.

Most of the time, we get so bogged down in what we don't like about our bodies, especially their appearance, that we miss what our bodies DO. I'll give you a couple of things I appreciate about my body. Then, I'd love to hear something about your body that you appreciate.

Be mindful to present examples that represent a spectrum of characteristics and physical abilities so as to be inclusive of those with disabilities. For example, you might say you appreciate your ability to breathe and to meditate when stressed. You might be grateful for how your body heals from illness and injuries. You might appreciate your arms because they allow you to hug your parent, partner, or best friend.

It's possible your client or a group member will express gratitude for an aspect of appearance. Because the purpose of this exercise is to generate body appreciation *beyond* appearance, try to reframe or redirect those comments with compassion. For instance, someone may like their toned arms: what do their arms make possible for them? Spend as much time as possible on this—it's valuable practice!

Between sessions, you'll ask your client or group members to try a writing exercise. This writing exercise is based on the intervention called **Expand Your Horizon**, originally developed by the brilliant researcher Jessica Alleva, PhD (Alleva et al., 2015). **Expand Your Horizon** consists of three writing exercises designed to increase body functionality appreciation. This intervention can yield lasting body image improvements (Alleva et al., 2015; Davies et al., 2022).

Ultimately, you want your client to complete all three exercises, but how you space them should depend on your client's capacity and any other exercises assigned. Body gratitude takes practice to cultivate, so if your client starts with the first exercise this week, be sure to assign the others in subsequent weeks. The handout starts with an introduction to the activity and contains a list of various body functions to help orient your clients to what body functionality encompasses. To begin, there are a few probing questions to generate ideas of what various body functions mean to your client. Take a moment to look over the first writing assignment with your client. How do they feel about the exercise? What do they imagine it'll be like to reflect on their body in this way?

The Harms of Self-Monitoring

If your client self-monitors their weight, body composition, or measurements, get curious about whether these behaviors help cultivate attunement to their bodily needs or whether they create *dis*connection. In Session 1, you asked your client to consider setting aside weight-loss goals and the practice of self-monitoring (e.g., of weight, eating, fitness). Focusing on external data naturally distracts from one's *internal* experience. And the act of monitoring for weight loss or weight maintenance implies the desire to be smaller or stay the same. Body acceptance is not about accepting one's body within a very narrowly defined range, but about allowing one's body to shift and change as needed. When your client is engaging in non-medically necessary self-monitoring practices[31], even small fluctuations are likely to disrupt attunement and lead to reactive behavior changes.

In Session 1, you had the option to do an exercise (**What If I Didn't Weigh Myself?**) directed at generating insight about how self-weighing specifically can disrupt intuitive eating. If your client chose to take a break from self-weighing, this is an ideal time to check in on how it's going. If your client wasn't ready yet, see if they'd be ready now by completing that exercise. Feel free to replace references to self-weighing with other forms of self-monitoring (e.g., calorie tracking) if more relevant for your client. If they want to take a break from the scale or consider not weighing themselves entirely, consider graduated exposure exercises to help them get there. I've had clients give their scales to family members, donate them, or make an art project from them. Some aren't quite ready to remove the scale from the house, so they ask a partner, roommate, or family member to hide it. When possible, getting the scale entirely out of one's home is best. When the scale remains accessible, it can be hard to resist the temptation to find it.

> Thin and straight-sized people almost always experience less friction from providers when advocating for themselves. This is especially true for white cisgender folks. Your client may not feel safe declining to be weighed. Support them in finding a way to get the care they need that minimizes harms. As a provider, you can be an advocate for your patient; for instance, I always try to get a release to speak with my clients' physicians so we can collaborate to provide high-quality care. In the past, I've specifically requested that my patients be weighed backwards and only when medically necessary, and that medical care providers center conversations around resources and lifestyle, not weight.

The Doctor's Office

Weigh-ins are so routine at the doctor's office that many of us just comply without considering that we have choices. I've worked with *many* people who avoided going to the doctor, *even when experiencing symptoms*, due to past negative—even discriminatory—experiences. Therefore, assess your client's comfort with going to the doctor. If going to the doctor is a source of stress, chat with them about their options. These are listed on the **Tips for Navigating Doctor Visits** handout, which I strongly recommend you provide to your clients.

Opposite Action: Treating the Body with Kindness

One additional approach your client can take toward body respect is engaging in intentional acts to take care of their body. When your client is feeling unkind toward their body, what is one

---

31 In limited circumstances, clients may have medically necessary reasons to self-monitor. For instance, patients with heart failure often weigh themselves regularly to monitor fluid accumulation.

Session 7: Body Respect 133

thing they could do to *nurture* it? Opposite action is a core DBT skill. It's helpful when we experience an intense emotion that compels us to engage in a behavior that may be destructive. Choosing to act in a way that is opposite of this urge—for example, mindful movement, taking a bath, cooking a delicious dinner, or painting one's nails—can help us rewire more adaptive ways of coping.

Step 5: Responding to Body Talk

Due to the cultural obsession with appearance and bodies, these topics come up *a lot* in conversation. Almost always, comments (positive or negative) reinforce weight stigma, gender norms, appearance ideals, and the importance of appearance to one's value. It's easy to understand why bashing someone else's body or appearance would be harmful, but positive comments can be harmful too. When someone loses weight, they almost always receive admiration and congratulations; yet there are many reasons a person may lose weight, including an eating disorder, serious illness, depression, or substance use. (When my mother was undergoing cancer treatment, her oncologist congratulated her on her quite unintentional weight loss.) Complimenting someone on their appearance reinforces its importance. Further, appearance and bodies change over time. If you're with a partner who constantly tells you they love your butt or your stomach, you might be afraid their attraction to you will fade if your body changes. For all these reasons, you want to help your client reduce their own body talk and learn how to respond when it comes up. Even with the firmest boundaries and the utmost vigilance, body talk is impossible to entirely avoid. Although most of my family and friends know that I won't participate in it, I still hear it in social settings, at work, and in public. It's good to help your clients practice how to navigate these situations.

There are many ways to respond to body talk depending on the context, including removing oneself from the situation, changing the conversation, or speaking up. Below is a two-part exercise. First, your client explores the *types* of comments that often come up and how they typically respond, then they come up with other ways they could respond. Then, you'll role-play responses to body talk. It can be challenging in the moment to have a quick response, especially when emotions are high. The goal of the role-play is to make these responses more accessible in the moment. Your client will also complete a between-session exercise to generate more ideas.

I recommend writing out responses to each part of this exercise, as it's helpful for your client to have something tangible they can refer to. If they have a list of possible responses to negative body talk, they can review it before going into a potentially triggering situation.

EXERCISE: Part 1—Options for Responding to Body Talk

1. **Body talk comes up a lot in conversations. As you work to change your relationship with your body, hearing comments about people's appearance and bodies can feel frustrating and even triggering. What kinds of comments do you hear people make?**

2. When these kinds of comments come up, how do you typically respond?

3. What ideas do you have about how to navigate these comments and conversations in the future?

   Allow your client or group members to generate ideas. Some that you may want to add are:

   - Stop personally commenting on the appearance and size of others' bodies, positively *or* negatively
   - Change the topic of conversation to one not involving appearance or eating/food
   - Model a comment in response that's aligned with one's values (e.g., responding to an appearance-based comment with one informed by body functionality appreciation or body neutrality)
   - Remove oneself from the situation
   - Set boundaries around these topics (e.g., asking a loved one to not comment on your body)

4. Speak up! If your client has the bandwidth to educate, they might choose to plant some seeds about weight bias.

EXERCISE: Part 2—Role-Play of Body Talk Responses

This exercise is especially fun in a group setting, but it works well in individual sessions, too As the facilitator, you can play the role of someone engaging in negative body talk, and your client can practice responding. Or you and your client can switch back and forth between roles. In a group setting, make sure everyone gets a chance to practice responding.

First, give an example so your client or group understands the activity (see below). In a group, I have the two leaders role-play together once to model the exercise:

Group Leader 1: These pants feel so tight. I've gained so much weight.

Group Leader 2: The fit of your pants has nothing to do with what an amazing person you are. Maybe we could go to the store and look for pants that make you feel good and comfortable.

OR: I love your style. Your pants look so cool with that shirt!

It's most helpful if clients or group members can practice responding to body talk that is salient to *them*. Ask them for body- or appearance-related comments they commonly hear or have heard recently. Write down their ideas. It's helpful to have a few of your own to add in case they have trouble thinking of comments.

In this exercise, it's crucial to redirect or reframe when your client's responses inadvertently reinforce weight stigma or are still appearance-based. For instance, if one of the comments is "I look so fat," responding with "You don't look fat" or "You're beautiful" reinforces the notion

Session 7: Body Respect

that "fat" equals bad or ugly. Your client can certainly reinforce all that they find beautiful about someone, including their sense of humor, creativity, and so on.

It's helpful to introduce this activity by noting, before beginning the role-play, that you will chat (either you and your client or as a group) about any comments that might reinforce weight stigma or appearance norms and then come up with some alternative comments that don't. When clients feel it's OK to be learning and growing, they're more likely to see these redirections as learning opportunities.

In a group setting, try to do at least one round where every group member gets a chance to practice. In an individual session, role-play a few comments. Then debrief on what it was like to do the exercise. Validate if clients found it challenging to generate responses—that's one of the primary reasons the exercise is worthwhile! Ask your client to take note of the different appearance and body-related comments they hear over the next week. Then ask them to write down the comments and their potential responses. It's totally OK if they struggle in the moment to respond. I've been doing this work for many years and I'd say I bat about .500. Sometimes I just stammer, stare blankly, or walk away. However, I always reflect on it later and think of what I *wish* I had said, which is so valuable in equipping me with responses in the future. My batting average is inching up!

Step 6: Social Media

Social media are now a part of most people's daily lives. In 2021, Pew Research Center estimated that seven in ten Americans use social media (Pew Research Center, 2021). And, although social media have some benefits, such as facilitating social interaction and connection (Gillespie-Smith et al., 2021; Naslund et al., 2020), there is a clear link between social media use and both body dissatisfaction and disordered eating risk (Harriger et al., 2023).

Social media are saturated with appearance-focused content, which engender social comparisons. Further, people often share idealized and filtered images of themselves and their lives. Influencers rely on high traffic and engagement for revenue and are paid by companies to promote their products. Therefore, people are increasingly exposed to products and wellness information not backed by science and that can even be dangerous. Perhaps most troubling is that social media companies now rely on algorithms that bias the content users see (Harriger et al., 2022). Unfortunately, these algorithms often have a rabbit hole effect, driving users into more niche and less moderated content. Your clients may be exposed to harmful content that is amplifying their body image and eating concerns and making healing harder. Social media literacy—learning about social media algorithms, the filtering and idealization of content, and the ubiquity of misinformation and paid content—is key for your client to be able to parse the content they view, including rejecting or avoiding content that threatens their body image (Tylka & Wood-Barcalow, 2015). If your client is a heavy social media user, talk to them about the apps they use, the types of accounts they follow, and their frequency of use. There are several steps your client can take to decrease the potential harms associated with social media use listed on the **Social Media Strategies** handout. Consider setting a goal around social media use for the next week.

Step 7: Between-Session Exercises and Closing

Your client has two primary exercises this week. First, they will be completing *at least* the first writing assignment from the **Expand Your Horizon** writing activity. The goal is to help your client cultivate gratitude for their body's functions, helping shift their body image so that appearance is no longer the primary way they relate to their body or measure its worth. Ask your client to bring the exercise with them to the next session if they're willing. In that session, you will ask if they would be willing to share a snippet of what they wrote.

The **Negative Body Talk** exercise involves your client taking note of the various appearance- and body-related comments they hear throughout the week. Regardless of how they responded in the moment, they will use this exercise to generate potential responses for when similar things come up in the future.

Finally, your client might set a goal to stop or reduce their self-weighing behavior or modify their social media use.

Closing

As always, close out the session by sharing something that hit home this week.

Session 7: Body Respect

Lengthening the Session

When we piloted this intervention, many participants wanted more time to talk about body image. If you have time to break this session into two, I highly recommend it! Lengthening this session could be particularly helpful for clients with:

- Body dysmorphic disorder
- High internalized weight bias
- Strong anti-fat attitudes
- A medical condition or disability that affects body image
- Heavy social media use
- Exposure to considerable negative body talk or anti-fat attitudes (e.g., loved ones who are dieting, or who work in a medical setting)
- Less experience talking about body image (it may take a couple of sessions to warm up)

To lengthen this session, I suggest:

- Spending the first session on Steps 2 and 3
- Spending the second session on Steps 4 and 6

Shortening the Session

If you have fewer than ten sessions with your client, this is one of the most important to include: whenever possible, I recommend not skipping this content! However, if body image is less salient to your client or you have less time, choose the content you think will be most relevant to your client. For instance, if your client is already savvy on weight science and fat liberation, you could skip the Step 2 introduction about body diversity and how bodies fight against attempts at weight suppression. Similarly, if your client is fairly body neutral or even body positive, you can skip Step 3 and you may not need to spend a lot of time on Step 4. I do suggest doing Step 5 (Responding to Body Talk), because everyone encounters it in their daily lives and it's good to have ideas on how to respond. Finally, if your client doesn't use social media, I still recommend at least briefly touching on social media literacy in case they use it in the future. However, you may not need to spend time detailing protective strategies for social media use.

CHAPTER 11

Session 8: Finding Joy in Movement

Session Outline

Step 1: Between-Session Exercises Debriefing

　Expand Your Horizon

　Negative Body Talk

Step 2: Exploring Terminology: Exercise vs. Movement

　Exercise: Exploring Terminology

Step 3: Overview of Intuitive Movement

　Exercise: Exploring My Relationship with Movement

　Introducing Intuitive Movement

　Handout: Types of Movement

　Exercise: Could Intuitive Movement Work for Me?

Step 4: Exploring Benefits of and Barriers to Movement

　Exercise: Exploring the Benefits of and Barriers to Intuitive Movement

　Handout: Barriers to Intuitive Movement

　Optional Exercise: Arguing for Intuitive Movement

Step 5: Compensatory, Compulsive, and Over-Exercise

　Optional Exercise and Handout: Maladaptive Movement Quiz & Reflection

Step 6: Between-Session Exercises & Closing

　Barriers to Intuitive Movement

　Movement Log & Reflection

　Optional: Maladaptive Movement Quiz & Reflection

Materials

Types of Movement

Barriers to Intuitive Movement

Movement Log & Reflection

Maladaptive Movement Quiz & Reflection (optional)

Session Aim

Although movement[32] can be joyful and nourishing, many people develop a fraught relationship with it. This makes sense given how movement is typically portrayed: media and healthcare providers bombard us with messages about the dangers of a sedentary lifestyle. Businesses and advertisers capitalize on this fearmongering to sell gym memberships, supplements, and workout gear replete with slogans like "No pain, no gain." Indeed, movement is often discussed in terms of its effects on calorie burn and/or body modification. Wellness influencers promote these products, which increases their allure and helps reinforce the messaging that only strenuous exercise "counts" as movement and the purpose of exercise is to burn off calories and/or change one's body. It's no wonder people often feel movement requires suffering and see it as a means to either change their body, burn off what they ate, or earn what they plan to eat. However, "fitspiration" images on social media *aren't* motivating: they're associated with poorer mood, lower self-esteem, and increased body dissatisfaction across genders (Fatt et al., 2019; Prichard et al., 2020). Further, fitspiration images appear to increase appearance-based motives for exercise, which are related to greater disordered eating (Tylka & Homan, 2015; Vartanian et al., 2012).

The ninth principle of intuitive eating is about developing a new perspective on and relationship with movement. Here are a few defining features:

- Broadening one's concept of what "counts" as movement (not just strenuous cardio or weight training)

- Finding forms of movement that feel good in one's body (which can vary day to day)

- Tuning in to what the body is communicating about its needs for type, duration, and frequency of movement

- Decoupling movement from body modification or calorie burn

Of course there's nuance. For instance, if a person is interested in increasing their cardiorespiratory fitness, they'll need to engage in activities that increase their heart rate, which can be uncomfortable but does *not* require exercising to the point of getting sick. And once a person no longer sees movement as a way to change how their body looks or to burn off calories, they'll be freer to consider what kind of movement their body is looking for that day. They can begin to consider how movement may benefit them, like increasing mobility, flexibility, cardiorespiratory fitness, and mood, or providing a source of mindful time to oneself each day. Movement can also create opportunities for building community and social connectedness. Therefore, the goal of this session is to help your client shift their relationship with movement and help them find ways to move their body that feel *nourishing* instead of punishing.

---

32 Throughout this chapter, I'll primarily use the word "movement" to refer to any form of physical activity or exercise. This choice of words is intentional; the term "exercise" has become laden with meaning and associations. When people hear "exercise," they may be likely to think of a narrow set of activities. "Movement" might encourage one to think more broadly. Further, because "movement" is a less common term, it's free of the negative associations that come with "exercise" or even "physical activity."

Additional Considerations and Potential Adaptations

Avoid ableist language when discussing movement. In individual sessions, you should have a good grasp on your client's relationship with movement and their ability status. In a group setting, don't assume everyone is fully able-bodied. Many folks have disabilities or chronic illnesses that are not obvious. It can feel profoundly lonely to be in a group or social setting where ability is assumed. Group members with disabilities or chronic illnesses will likely miss the opportunity to explore and develop their own relationship with movement. Movement will look different for everyone, but especially for folks who have physical or capacity limitations. For instance, someone with a back injury may not be able to go for a jog but might benefit from connecting with a physical therapist or doing strength or mobility training. Or, someone with fibromyalgia or chronic fatigue syndrome might find benefit from gentle walks or stretching, and will likely have to modify depending on their symptoms on any given day.

Athletes will often have a different and more complex relationship with movement than nonathletes. Athletes are often encouraged to push past discomfort in pursuit of specific goals. And increasing cardiovascular fitness and strength of course requires effort, which can be uncomfortable. Pushing through some discomfort during movement isn't inherently a problem. Yet with athletes it can be a fine line. Often the internal or external pressure to improve or to reach a goal can motivate them to push past injury, illness, or signs of overtraining. Further, as mentioned in Chapter 2, some sports and athletic activities pressure athletes to obtain a lean-body composition to aid performance or competition, which can lead to overtraining and under-nourishing. So some of the content in this session will need to be reframed when working with athletes. You'll likely focus on their intentions for movement (including their athletic goals), how much they're listening to their body to avoid overtraining or under-nourishing, the benefits they derive from movement, and any barriers they experience to engaging in their sport in a way that is nourishing to their mental and physical health.

Finally, people will differ in their access to movement for other reasons, including time, finances, housing, stigma, and safety. Some folks will have less time to engage in movement. Others will be limited in the types of movement they can afford (e.g., memberships, equipment). Many fitness spaces can be discriminatory for folks in large, Black, Brown, or disabled bodies. Finally, some people live in neighborhoods that are not safe for outdoor recreation. If any of these factors are true for your client, you'll need to brainstorm how movement might look for *them*.

Considerations for Group Interventions

In a group setting, people will likely have different needs around movement. Some folks may be looking to increase their movement or find new forms of movement that feel good in their bodies. Some folks may need to cut back or take a break from their usual activities entirely (especially those who engage in compensatory or compulsive exercise or who are overtrained). Be inclusive in your language so that members don't feel othered, or don't miss out on this opportunity to work on their relationship with movement.

Step 1: Between-Session Exercises Debriefing

You asked your client to complete at least the first of three **Expand Your Horizon** writing exercises. These exercises involve writing, continuously and unfiltered, for 15 minutes about functions of the body one appreciates. The goal of this exercise was to help your client begin to change how they view their body. Check in on how this exercise went for your client. How challenging was it? What insights did they gain? Do they think continuing this gratitude writing practice will be helpful? It's unlikely that completing one exercise radically changed your client's body image, which has likely developed over many years. Attitude change doesn't happen overnight! If your client just completed the first exercise, encourage them to complete the second in the upcoming week. I also like to ask my client or group members if they'd be willing to share any piece of their writing. This is completely optional, but it can be meaningful.

For the **Negative Body Talk** exercise, your client noted the various appearance- and body-related comments they heard throughout the week, and considered potential responses they could use in the future (especially if they didn't respond as they wanted in the moment). What types of comments did they hear? How did they respond? How might they want to respond in the future? Feel free to workshop some responses with them in session, keeping in mind that directly challenging body talk is not always the safest option. Sometimes the best options are to walk away, change the conversation, or simply ignore the comment.

Step 2: Exploring Terminology: Exercise Versus Movement

In this session, you will bury the lead. That is, before introducing what intuitive movement is, you'll get your client thinking about their current views on movement by exploring the terminology they use to describe it. This exploration isn't intended to change your client's language—they can certainly use whatever words they want! Rather, it may provide insights on whether their current conceptualization of movement is limited.

If your client is an athlete, you may want to move directly to Step 3, where they can explore their relationship with their sport or activities of choice.

EXERCISE: Exploring Terminology

1. **When you think of the term "exercise," what activities come to mind?**

    This question should give you a clue as to how your client views movement. Do they mention a narrow range of activities (e.g., running, gym cardio, strength training) or do they conceptualize exercise more broadly?

2. **What comes up for you when you think about the word "exercise"? Does it evoke any particular reactions or emotions?**

Your clients' reactions to exercise may be complex. One may view exercise as punishing or a dreaded obligation. The term may elicit feelings of guilt or shame. Others may have a positive relationship with exercise, and the term may elicit feelings of excitement or enthusiasm. Some folks may experience a combination of reactions, so embrace the dialectic and affirm your clients' feelings!

3. **Now, think about the word "movement." What activities come to mind? Does the word evoke any specific reactions or emotions?**

    The goal of this question is to explore whether "movement" might be a more palatable term than "exercise." When they think of movement, do they envision a broader range of activities?

4. **What differences did you notice between the terms? Does one word resonate more than the other?**

    There are no right or wrongs here! However, if the term "exercise" evokes negative reactions or a restricted range of activities for your client, they may consider that using the word "movement" could change how they view moving their body. How we think about movement is powerful; indeed, CBT is based on the idea that our thoughts shape our feelings and our feelings shape our behaviors. If we think about movement in a different way, it could change how we *feel* about it, and thus what movement we *do*.

The goal of this exploration of terminology is to get your client thinking about their current perspective on movement so they're ready to dig into their own relationship with it.

Step 3: Overview of Intuitive Movement

Almost everyone knows that movement is "good" for you. Yet, the actual purpose and benefits of movement can get lost in the mainstream messaging around it. Exercise can begin to feel like an obligation, something done to burn calories, or something that involves suffering, which is rarely motivating. People crave autonomy and choice; feeling like something is "required" can remove the enjoyment. Further, if you fully expect movement to be boring, painful, or otherwise unenjoyable, you're less likely to want to do it. Some folks will push past the discomfort or feeling of obligation but may still engage in movement they don't enjoy or that doesn't align with their body's needs. Does this sound familiar? It's remarkably like dieting! To start, you'll ask your client to explore their *current* relationship with movement.

EXERCISE: Exploring My Relationship with Movement

1. **What is your current relationship with movement like? For instance, does it feel like something you want to do, have to do, or a bit of both?**

2. **What are your reasons for engaging in movement? What are the outcomes you are hoping or expecting to get?**

3. **Try to think of a time when you engaged in movement out of a sense of obligation, or when you chose an activity because you were concerned about your eating or body image. How did exercising for those reasons affect your motivation? What about your enjoyment of the activity?**

   Some people might have felt *more* motivated to be active when they felt obligated. Still, it's important to explore the experience of that exercise. Was it enjoyable? Rejuvenating?

4. **What types of activities did you choose when exercise felt like an obligation, or when you were concerned about your eating or body image?**

Introducing Intuitive Movement

Now, you want to introduce the concept of intuitive movement, communicating that, ultimately, intuitive movement is an ongoing process that involves: (1) global and day-to-day observations on the types of movement their body seems to need and/or enjoy; and (2) mindfully attending to how their body feels before, during, and after activity.

Globally, your client may notice their body could benefit from added stamina, strength, flexibility, and/or mobility, or they may be interested in how movement could improve their mental health. Some days they may notice they feel a bit sore or stiff and think some stretching or yoga would feel good in their body. Other days, they may feel energetic and want to do a higher intensity activity.

During the activity, clients would be paying attention to when their body is reaching its satiation point, and would stop if they feel exhausted or sick. Afterward, they would pay attention to both the short- and long-term effects. For instance, they might notice immediately after engaging in movement that their muscles feel looser and their mood is boosted. Long-term, they might notice their mood has been more stable, and they feel recharged after consistently taking time to themselves.

Intuitive movement also includes choosing activities based on how much your client enjoys them and whether they align with your client's needs, rather than how many calories the activities will burn or how much they might change how your client's body looks. For instance, your client may realize they like team-based sports (e.g., soccer), but don't particularly enjoy endurance cardio. Or perhaps they enjoy long, solo bike rides and social time after.

Movement should be properly nourished, and not done to burn off or "earn" food (a sign of compensatory exercise). Finally, the movement needs of those with differences in interoceptive awareness may involve more structure (e.g., setting a movement schedule), an emphasis on enjoyment, and avoiding exercises that are physiologically aversive.

For the following exercise, you'll guide your client through thinking about whether intuitive movement might work for them. It'll be helpful to have the **Types of Movement** list handy for this exercise.

EXERCISE: Could Intuitive Movement Work for Me?

1. **Now that you've heard a bit about intuitive movement, what comes up when you think about approaching movement in this way?**

2. **What types of activities might you choose if your choice was guided by enjoyment or goals not related to appearance or weight, like endurance, strength, or mental health?**

    Here, you can provide the **Types of Movement** list to help your client brainstorm the types of activities that might appeal to them.

3. **Where might you want to be active? For instance, would you want to do home-based workouts, to go to the gym, and/or move outdoors? Would you want to engage in movement alone or with others?**

    These questions are intended to help your client think about the contexts in which they'll enjoy or benefit from movement most. Most likely, they'll sometimes want to move outside, sometimes at home, sometimes alone, and sometimes with others.

    As mentioned, not everyone has access to safe spaces for outdoor recreation, and many gyms are unsafe spaces for those in marginalized bodies. Additionally, movement is inherently bound by one's resources, including money and time.

4. **How might approaching movement in this way affect the frequency or duration of your exercise?**

    This question can apply to clients who desire more movement in their life *or* to those who could benefit from less. You don't want to suggest that movement is inherently better or more desirable when it is more frequent or of longer duration, since clients' movement needs are highly contextual. People often get fixated on data (such as step count) and goals driven by external factors (such as physical activity app-based recommendations). Because such fixations can lead one to engage in movement that is out of alignment with their body's needs, intuitive eating principles do not lead to explicit recommendations for how often or how long people engage in movement.

The purpose of this exercise was to get curious without judgment, and to begin to explore what intuitive movement might look like for your client. It'll be different for everyone and might change from week to week. The point is to affirm that movement *does not* have to be an obligation, a punishment, or unpleasant.

Step 4: Exploring Benefits of and Barriers to Movement

Now that your client has begun to explore what moving more intuitively might look like for them, it's time to consider the potential benefits of and barriers to such movement. If your client realizes that approaching movement more intuitively might benefit their quality of life or better align with their values, their motivation to make that shift will likely increase. However, to actually start shifting their relationship with movement, it's crucial to consider potential roadblocks. Have the **Barriers to Intuitive Movement** quiz handy to refer to in the second part of this discussion.

For clients who are athletes, you'll want to focus specifically on the benefits they derive from participating in their sport(s) of choice and any barriers to approaching their sport in a more intuitive way.[33]

EXERCISE: Exploring the Benefits of and Barriers to Intuitive Movement

1. **After exploring what intuitive movement might look like for you, what do you think some of the short-term benefits would be?**

    Short-term benefits can be gleaned whether your client is looking to engage in more, less, or different types of movement. Benefits might include positive mood, feelings of self-efficacy, strength, flexibility, stamina, sleep, increased social connectedness, or improved mental clarity. Athletes might notice improved performance. Try to redirect if your client or group mentions appearance or weight-based reasons for engaging in movements. Some may feel that reducing their weight will improve their mobility (e.g., reduced knee pain). In that case, you could reinforce that knee pain can be reduced independent of weight loss via strength, flexibility, and mobility training.

2. **What about some of the long-term benefits?**

    Some of the short-term benefits may be long-term, as well. For instance, your client may feel increased social connectedness through more time spent engaging in movement with others *or* having more time for cultivating relationships rather than working out. Athletes may experience less injury or illness, increasing the quality and longevity of their sport participation. Consistent movement over time can benefit mental health, bone density, and cardiovascular function, and reduce health risks like cognitive decline, certain types of cancer, heart disease, and insulin resistance.

---

[33] It is certainly possible your client has a healthy relationship with their sport or movement already; if so, you can focus more on the benefits they have observed and any barriers that could threaten the positive relationship they have cultivated.

3. **Now, what could get in the way of approaching movement more intuitively?**

    You can provide the **Barriers to Intuitive Movement** quiz to guide discussion. If your client is unsure what their main barriers are, you might start by asking what factors may have led them to engage in movement that *wasn't* intuitive previously. For instance, does your client still follow fitness influencers on social media or have friends who approach movement in an *un*intuitive way? Some folks may lack self-efficacy. For instance, they may be interested in beginning weight training, but are unsure how to use the equipment. Or, they may have experienced discrimination when working out or in fitness spaces and are unsure which activities and spaces are safe. Others may work long hours, have limited financial resources, or have care-giving responsibilities, all of which make it challenging to fit in and prioritize movement. Finally, your client may not wish to change anything about their current relationship with movement. That's OK! In this case, you could ask what might reduce the peace they have around movement. Understanding real and potential barriers can help you explore together how to overcome them.

4. **Thinking about the barriers we just identified, what would you say are the top two? What ideas do you have for how to overcome them?**

    In a group setting, you can allow your group members to think on their own before brainstorming as a group. Keep in mind that because being less active is stigmatized, those who are more active may feel more confident to speak up in the group.

    In individual sessions, help your client come up with solutions. For instance, if your client feels like taking time for movement is selfish, ask them to consider whether taking that time for themselves could help them recharge and be more present for their loved ones. For clients who need home-based workouts (and have internet or cell phone access), discuss seeking out online videos that can give them access to dance classes, yoga, cycling, and more. And if your client currently has an adaptive relationship with movement, it's worth naming what factors make that possible.

This week, your client will work on addressing one of their **modifiable** intuitive movement barriers. Again, this won't necessarily be a barrier to engaging in movement altogether. For some, it could be addressing something that gets in the way of moving in a way that is aligned with their body's needs. Some barriers will of course not be modifiable. If your client doesn't feel comfortable engaging in movement in their neighborhood or a gym space, you can consider together some ways to move in their home. For clients with busy schedules (e.g., multiple jobs, caregiving responsibilities), it may be most important to prioritize sleep. Create one **specific** goal for this week. For instance, do they notice they tend to work out for a set duration of time or do a specific type of movement, regardless of how their body feels? Perhaps their goal could be to do at least one session *mindfully*; that is, tuning in to the experiencing and noting when their body is ready to stop. It could also mean choosing a different type of movement that their body may enjoy or desire more.

Additionally, your client will be logging some information about their movement over the week on the **Movement Log & Reflection**. The purpose of this tracking is *not* to set rigid parameters around the type, frequency, duration, or intensity of their movement (unless that's

Session 8: Finding Joy in Movement

needed…more in a moment!). Rather, it's to log their *experience* of movement throughout the week. What forms of movement did they gravitate toward? Was it challenging to choose activities for reasons other than calorie burn or body modification? If they engaged in movement, how would they rate its *quality* (pleasant, unpleasant, neutral)? Finally, there are reflection questions designed to generate insights and identify patterns (e.g., do they enjoy solo or social movement?).

Your client may benefit from setting goals around the type, duration, and/or frequency of their movement. This could be especially true in the context of busy schedules or neurodivergence. I have worked with college students with ADHD, for example, who benefit from structured activity. This may sound like an oxymoron, but there can be flexibility built into structure! For instance, if your client sets the goal of attending a fitness class in the morning, but then has a bad night of sleep, they can choose to sleep in and reschedule the class for later in the day or week. What you want your client to avoid is becoming so fixated on their schedule that they override their bodily needs or generate distress or impairment.

OPTIONAL EXERCISE: Arguing for Intuitive Movement

Time permitting, you can include an exercise where you or your group leader play the role of someone who views movement as punishing or compensatory (exercise that's inherently unpleasant or done to earn or make up for eating). Have your client or a group member explain and make an argument for *intuitive* movement. This exercise is especially helpful when you perceive your client's perception of exercise is deeply ingrained and they would benefit from more practice perceiving movement differently.

Step 5: Compensatory, Compulsive, and Over-Exercise

Public health campaigns are often aimed at encouraging people to move *more*. Extreme forms of exercise are often applauded or even encouraged. Many fitness spaces have slogans and advertisements encouraging people to push through pain, messages which are often reinforced via media (*especially* social media). Although people can usually readily name the consequences of an inactive lifestyle, there seems to be no upper limit on the amount of movement considered acceptable or "healthy." Fitness tracking apps and devices reinforce this idea, continually adjusting your step goals upward with seemingly no ceiling—and they track your movement trends and send notifications when you've been less active than usual. You don't even have to opt in to these devices—chances are your phone is already tracking your steps! Therefore, some of your clients may not realize that there *is* such a thing as unhealthy exercise.

Movement is considered "disordered" when it's done in an excessive, compulsive, or compensatory manner. For some, disordered exercise may mean exercising for long periods of time or exercising very intensely. For others, the time or intensity might seem "normal," but the intentions are not healthy. Many folks who engage in maladaptive exercise have rigid rules that are distressing to break, and obeying them can lead to skipping social activities or working out when sick or injured. Others might exercise in a compensatory way, either to make up for eating or to "earn" something they plan to eat. These types of movement are harmful physically *and* mentally. Not only can you harm your body by pushing it past its limits or not fueling it properly, you also miss out on the many benefits that come from moving more intuitively.

The **Maladaptive Movement Quiz** and accompanying reflection questions are included to help your client determine if they're exercising in a maladaptive way. Time permitting, you can go through the results in session and use that information to set goals for the week. Some clients may need to take a break or majorly scale back their movement to allow their body or mind to recover. This can generate considerable anxiety for some clients who may be concerned about losing fitness or their body changing. However, taking a break or scaling back may benefit their performance in the longer term because it will provide the body a chance to reset. Perhaps they could incorporate some new, gentler activities (e.g., yoga). If your client's anxiety is particularly high, it'll likely be useful to return to the graduated exposure exercises from Session 3.

This exercise is **optional** *if* it's clear your client doesn't have issues with maladaptive movement. However, in a group setting I recommend including this quiz as a between-session exercise because maladaptive movement may be an issue for some members.

Step 6: Between-Session Exercises and Closing

Your client has two closely related exercises for this week. First, they'll work on reducing one barrier to intuitive movement and reflect on this experience using the **Barriers to Intuitive Movement** handout. Additionally, they'll log their movement on the **Movement Log & Reflection** handout, *provided* their goal is not to take a break from movement. If they are taking a break, they'll log and reflect on what it's like to rest or move their bodies in gentler ways. In general, the handout is designed to help your client increase their attunement to their *unique* movement needs. There are no specific goals on how many times they log over the week, as every client's needs will be different. Finally, if your client engages in maladaptive movement, you'll provide the **Maladaptive Movement Quiz & Reflection** to complete over the week.

Closing

Close out by sharing something that resonated with you and your client or group members from this session.

Lengthening the Session

If time and resources permit, this session can be expanded into two. Lengthening this session could be particularly helpful for clients who:

- Are athletes
- Engage in maladaptive exercise
- Have a history of discriminatory physical activity experiences
- Have a medical condition or disability that limits accessibility of movement
- Have limited time or financial resources

To lengthen this session, I suggest:

- Spending the first session on Steps 2 and 3
- Spending the second session on Steps 4 and 5

Shortening the Session

You may be able to shorten or skip this session if your client has an adaptive or peaceful relationship with movement. Conversely, you may choose to skip this session if movement is not currently accessible to your client or is not a priority. If your client is on movement restrictions, you may want to revisit this topic later.

How you shorten this session will depend on your client. If your client already engages in intuitive movement, you may want to jump to Step 4 and consider ways to keep that adaptive relationship going. Conversely, if your client has an adaptive relationship with exercise but is unfamiliar with the concept of intuitive movement, you may want to introduce it and explore the ways they are currently practicing it. You can skip the discussion on terminology if it's not relevant for your client.

CHAPTER 12

Session 9: Gentle Nutrition

Session Outline

Step 1: Between-Session Exercises Debriefing

    Barriers to Intuitive Movement

    Movement Log & Reflection

    Optional: Maladaptive Movement Quiz & Reflection

Step 2: Overview of Gentle Nutrition

    Exercise and Handout: Body–Food Choice Congruence

Step 3: Play Food (or Just…Food)

    Exercise and Handout: Rethinking Terminology

Step 4: Am I Ready for Gentle Nutrition?

    Exercise and Handout: Am I Ready for Gentle Nutrition?

Step 5: The Pursuit of Progress over Perfection

    Exercise: Part 1—How Does Shame Serve Me?

    Handout: Patience and Progress

    Exercise: Part 2—Practicing Self-Compassion and Curiosity

    Optional Exercise and Handout: What Is Food For?

Step 6: Between-Session Exercises and Closing

    Body–Food Choice Congruence

    Patience and Progress

Materials

Body–Food Choice Congruence

Rethinking Terminology

Am I Ready for Gentle Nutrition?

What Is Food For?

Patience and Progress

Session Aim

Many people want to eat "healthy,"[34] but their motivations for this are complex and challenging to disentangle. Although many likely *do* want to eat in ways that will make their bodies and minds feel good, reduce disease risk, and aid longevity, they also likely feel *pressure* to do so, given that "healthy" eating has become almost a moral imperative. Many may also hope that eating "healthy" will ultimately change how their bodies look. Yet, these days it's hard to know what "healthy" eating even means. Despite the latest dieting trends and the confident claims of endless influencers, there is no one "right" or "best" way to eat. As discussed in Session 4, humans evolved in many different climates with varying food availability. Because our bodies are smart, they adapted in response. There is no one dietary pattern that has demonstrated itself to be superior for health over the others.[35]

I get the desire to find the "best" way to eat. I can see the appeal of being told that if you eat XYZ at these times in these amounts, you'll feel great, avoid diseases, and live a long time (although I can also see how that could remove some joy from eating). Yet, "healthy" eating is highly contextual, and pleasure is important. Sometimes, broccoli, rice, and salmon will be a highly nutritious meal that aligns with someone's needs. But certainly, that meal isn't "healthy" if someone is allergic to fish. Ice cream may be the "healthiest" option when one has avoided it for years and is trying now to make peace with ice cream. Sometimes, someone's body may need extra iron, sodium, fat, or fiber. Other times, someone may be hypoglycemic, and sugar is vital for stabilizing insulin levels. Therefore, the goal of this session is to help your client move away from rigid perceptions of "healthy" eating and learn how to gauge what is right for their body at any given time. A crucial step toward this goal is ensuring your client is *ready* for this exploration; clients with a lingering diet mentality will need to do further work on addressing that before proceeding to gentle nutrition.

If your client is still working to make peace with food, I urge you to start with Step 4, Am I Ready for Gentle Nutrition? This exercise will help them identify the motivations for their food choices and elucidate whether continued work on earlier principles is needed prior to embarking upon gentle nutrition. In this case, you can introduce the concept of gentle nutrition, but perhaps spend the remainder of the session focusing on principles where they could use additional practice and support.

---

34   Throughout this chapter, I will put the words "healthy" and "unhealthy" in quotations. Ultimately, when working with clients, I avoid using these terms because they have become so opaque and laden with other meanings. Therefore, I tend to say "nutritious" when some sort of descriptor is needed, but we'll get into the nuances more throughout this chapter.

35   Although some research suggests the Mediterranean diet may be favorable for health long-term, the diet itself remains poorly demarcated.

Additional Considerations and Potential Adaptations

Gentle nutrition will look different for your clients depending on the availability and accessibility of nutritious foods for them. Many people cannot access or afford fresh produce, or do not live close to a grocery store. Therefore, it's essential that these factors are considered when you explore how your client might practice gentle nutrition. For instance, if your client is interested in increasing their fruit or vegetable consumption, it's important to dispel myths that canned and frozen produce are less nutritious. If affordability is a concern, investigate local resources for food assistance, including food pantries and community-supported agriculture. For therapists who have clients with medically necessary dietary considerations (e.g., diabetes), it's best to collaborate with a registered dietitian.

Neurodivergent folks, especially autistic people, may have a limited range of foods they eat, and some of these may be labeled in the mainstream as "unhealthy." Yet, these foods may enable an autistic person to get their nutritional needs met. The focus should always be on ensuring adequate nutrition: if certain "healthy" foods are unappealing or aversive to your client, they don't need to eat them![36] Let your client lead the way here. Are there any changes they want to make in the types of foods they eat? How are the foods they currently eat sitting on their stomach? How are their energy levels, mood, and sleep? Are there perhaps some adjustments to be made to help them feel better physically? Are there any foods they're interested in trying or incorporating more often?

As your client is exploring gentle nutrition, including how different foods feel in their bodies, they may be tempted to overgeneralize from single experiences. For instance, I've lost count of the number of people who've told me that carbs make them feel sluggish (I blame this at least partially on diet culture) and who have concluded they should limit or avoid them altogether. Now, don't get me wrong, it's entirely possible that someone has experienced sluggishness after eating a carb-dominant meal. Yet, context is *crucial*. There are so many questions to consider. What else did they eat? How long had it been since they'd eaten? How long until they ate again? Were they hydrated? How have they been sleeping? How well have they been nourishing themselves generally? Are they under a lot of stress? I could go on and on. The point is: It's entirely possible that several factors contributed to feeling sluggish and the solution isn't always to cut the food out completely.

There may be some foods that consistently don't sit well with your client—for instance, they may notice beans almost always make them gassy. For that reason, they may choose to avoid them most of the time, and approach eating them with intention. For instance, I love queso dip, but know if I eat it in large quantities, my digestive system will not be happy. So when I choose to eat queso, I opt for a smaller serving and eat it alongside foods that *do* sit well on my stomach. Throughout this session, encourage your client to consider the full context—and to be on the lookout for diet culture sneaking in.

---

36 If your client eats a restricted range of foods, assess for distress or impairment. Does food avoidance generate more consequences than it solves? Could your client's distress be ameliorated with reintroduction? Or, has your client learned what foods work for them, and thus eating a restricted range of foods *decreases* distress?

Session 9: Gentle Nutrition

> ### Considerations for Group Interventions
>
> Perhaps more than in any other session, your group members will have varying levels of both readiness for gentle nutrition and interoceptive awareness and accuracy. Whenever group members differ, opportunities are ripe for both learning *and* social comparison. It's easy for folks to compare themselves to group members who are farther along in feeling ready for gentle nutrition. But these aren't fair comparisons: each group member has unique life experiences, skills, challenges, and needs. Gentle nutrition will look different for each person. Folks who have differences in interoception may prioritize foods that minimize gastrointestinal upset or are palatable, facilitating sufficient intake. Others may have increased interoceptive accuracy and thus greater ability to identify what foods will feel best in their body at any given time. Finally, others may have the capacity to develop their interoceptive skills, but just aren't ready yet—and it's a strength, *not* a weakness to identify that. Therefore, be mindful of these dynamics throughout this session, being sure to validate and normalize each person's unique needs and strengths.

Step 1: Between-Session Exercises Debriefing

This week your client was asked to try to reduce one modifiable barrier to intuitive movement, and to make notes on the **Barriers to Intuitive Movement** handout. Some clients may have reduced a barrier that impedes movement altogether, whereas for others it could've involved shifting toward movement that is more aligned with their needs. Some clients may be attempting to take a break from or reduce their movement. Check in on how it went to reduce a barrier to intuitive movement. If it went well, you may consider addressing another barrier over the next week. If your client encountered challenges, explore together how they may address these challenges moving forward. It's also possible there is another more pressing barrier to address. Your client was asked to log their movement over the week, paying special attention to their physical, emotional, and mental experience before, during, and after using the **Movement Log & Reflection**. What did they notice? Was it challenging to choose what movement would feel good in their body and be enjoyable? Did they try any new activities? How do they want to approach movement in the next week?

The **Maladaptive Movement Quiz & Reflection** was optional, depending on your client's needs. If your client completed this, what do they think about their results? If your client is engaging in maladaptive movement behaviors, it's likely they will have complex feelings about shifting their approach to movement. Remember the fear-avoidance cycle introduced in Session 3? It's likely that your client's maladaptive exercise behaviors are serving a similar function of temporarily reducing anxiety and providing a sense of relief. It may be useful to walk through the short- and long-term outcomes of such behaviors with your client. How would these compare to the short- and long-term effects of movement that is more intuitive? Intuitive movement may not provide the same powerful anxiety relief in the short term. Yet in the long term, and especially in conjunction with the other intuitive eating principles, your client is likely to notice increased quality of life and lower anxiety, thus reducing the need for maladaptive exercise altogether. What's one step they could take this week toward intuitive movement?

In a group setting, you may want to spend less time on group members sharing their individual experiences (as hearing about maladaptive exercise could be triggering for some), and instead lead them through an exercise where they reflect on the short- and long-term costs and benefits of each approach to movement. You can then process as a group and speak generally about costs and benefits without getting into details of each group member's own exercise behaviors.

Step 2: Overview of Gentle Nutrition

People often view intuitive eating as an approach that ignores nutrition—but this is not the case! Intuitive eating is instead about working to dismantle our diet culture–laden beliefs *before* considering nutrition in one's food choices. When we are entrapped in diet culture, nutrition-related eating decisions are often guided by cultural notions about "good" and "bad" foods rather than our own experiences and bodily needs. Body–food choice congruence is the essence of gentle nutrition. Put simply, body–food choice congruence is about noticing how different foods feel in the body and using those data to guide future eating decisions. For instance, someone practicing gentle nutrition is basing their food choices on body functioning, performance, health, AND pleasure. They may also integrate nutrition-related science into their food choices, for example, if they're looking to increase their iron or protein intake. However, I encourage folks to approach gentle nutrition experientially, not purely cognitively. For instance, what do they notice happens to their energy or mood when they increase their consumption of iron-rich foods?

Gentle nutrition is, crucially, the tenth principle of intuitive eating; your client needed to first deconstruct where their beliefs about food came from and learn to tune in to their body's needs. Otherwise, they'd be likely to approach gentle nutrition by defaulting to cultural prescriptions about how they "should" eat, which would have kept them firmly rooted in diet culture. Hopefully, at this point, your client has come to view foods as morally and emotionally neutral. That is, your client understands they're not a better person if they choose to eat broccoli instead of ice cream. If your client has reached this point, they're likely ready to consider the health benefits of various foods and incorporate that information into their eating decisions.

Sometimes when people first stop dieting and start making peace with food, they don't want to eat the things they made themselves eat when they were micromanaging their eating. These foods may have become aversive; for instance, if they frequently made themselves eat a salad when they really wanted to share pizza with friends, it may feel punishing to choose a salad. Over time, your client will likely want to reincorporate *some* of these foods. However, this should happen naturally and not be forced into any schedule or program. Foods that were previously off-limits will be novel for a while, but that excitement will return to normal levels with habituation and trust these foods will not be restricted again. It'll get easier with time for your client to eat these to satisfaction. Certain foods will likely stay exciting, and that's OK! I eat chocolate every day, but I still get excited when someone offers me some. We don't judge dogs for getting excited about treats, so why do we judge ourselves for finding pleasure in eating?

Session 9: Gentle Nutrition

EXERCISE: Body–Food Choice Congruence

Your client may not be sure where to start when it comes to gentle nutrition. Therefore, the **Body–Food Choice Congruence** worksheet contains questions they can consider before and after eating. To get your client used to thinking about food in this way, you'll practice in session. Practicing together is especially helpful because you can help your client think contextually and spot areas where diet culture may be seeping in.

Ask your client to think of **two** recent eating experiences; one where they felt satisfied and good in their body and another where they noticed they were unsatisfied or didn't feel good physically. I like to start with the less positive experience so that you close out the activity by discussing a time when your client was practicing gentle nutrition (even if unknowingly).

As always, this activity should be guided with openness, curiosity, and compassion. If your client notices that a recent fast-food meal didn't make them feel good physically, they may default to feeling shame. Yet, choosing to eat fast food is *not* a moral choice, nor does one suboptimal experience mean fast food doesn't have a place in gentle nutrition.

1. **Think back to a recent experience when you didn't feel good in your body after eating. What do you remember about how you felt physically?**

    Consider energy levels, indigestion, heartburn, mental clarity, mood, or how satisfying or filling the foods were.

2. **What did you like or not like about how the foods you ate made you feel?**

    Here you're attempting to get at the quality of the experience. For instance, maybe your client noticed the food tasted really good, but it wasn't satisfying.

3. **Was this experience typical of how you feel when you eat these foods, or was it different?**

    Help your client consider the context so they're not tempted to overgeneralize the experience. For instance, they may have noticed that eating a donut for breakfast didn't sit well on their stomach and left them unsatisfied and hungry an hour later. Yet perhaps a donut paired with yogurt and fruit would provide a totally different experience. Or perhaps your client notices they experience digestive discomfort whenever they eat sugar-free candy, which could mean they don't tolerate sugar alcohols very well.

4. **How long do these foods tend to stay with you? Do they provide quick or lasting energy?**

    Foods that provide lasting energy are not always the best option! For instance, if your client has dinner plans in an hour but is meal-hungry now, a lighter food that provides quick energy (e.g., simple carbohydrates) may be the best choice. Alternatively, if your client is working a long shift where they'll be on their feet, they'll need something substantial that will provide lasting energy and satiety.

Now repeat these questions, focusing on your client's recent positive eating experiences. Make sure to highlight and affirm the ways your client was practicing gentle nutrition.

Step 3: Play Food (or Just...Food)

This section is quick, but I think it's important.

Language matters. It constructs our reality. Some folks may roll their eyes when terminology evolves, but there is a reciprocal process between how we talk about things and how we perceive them. If we repeatedly hear and refer to certain foods as "junk," then we will likely view these foods as disposable and of little value. Yet, for some folks, "junk" foods are what is accessible. And many of the foods labeled "junk" are delicious! It is truer and more productive to acknowledge that foods vary in their nutritional content and density. Some foods are higher in protein, others are higher in fat. Some are packed with important micronutrients, others aren't. Yet, all foods ultimately contain *some* nutritional value. Ice cream has fat, protein, and sugar, a combination that can give both satiety and satisfaction and provide quick energy. Potato chips have sodium, a crucial electrolyte, and fat. If a person were starving, they wouldn't turn away these foods. Why? Because these foods would keep them alive.

There is certainly cause to critique food and beverage companies, food marketing, the food lobby, and food-related public policies.[37] But these are *systemic* issues, not problems your clients have the responsibility to fix. If your client has access to and can afford a variety of nutritious foods, and notices that eating these foods tends to make them feel better physically and mentally, awesome! But you may work with clients who can't access or afford fresh produce, or who rely on packaged or convenience foods to meet their nutritional needs. These clients should not feel guilt because the foods they're eating are considered "junk." If you have worked in this field long enough, you know that villainizing or moralizing foods does more harm than good. Being shamed about your food choices isn't motivating or helpful.

Even if a food is less nutrient-dense, it still has its place. If your client repeatedly prioritized nutritional content over taste or satisfaction, eating would probably get pretty boring. Eating should also be enjoyable and even fun! Tribole and Resch (2017) note that people need fun foods like they need weekends, vacations, and breaks. If we're singularly focused on nutrition above all else, we might miss the joy in eating. As humans, we're primed to celebrate with food. We commemorate another year around the sun with cake, enjoy nice dinners on anniversaries, commune and feast with loved ones on holidays, and punctuate a meal with something sweet. Sorry, but never once have I wanted to celebrate a milestone or achievement with raw broccoli (and I love broccoli!).

Therefore, the next exercise is designed to get your client thinking about language and how it might shape their attitudes toward food. Your client might like the idea of switching up terminology from "junk" foods to "play" foods. However, tread with caution. For some clients, these foods are what is most accessible and affordable, and the term "play" could seem patronizing or dismissive. Ultimately, "play" foods are just food. You do want to encourage your client to move away from referring to these foods with a negative label, but whether they need their own

---

37 Yes, there is rising concern that ultra-processed foods may override interoceptive signaling and lead people to eat past satiety. Additionally, these foods often are not nutritionally complete. Villainizing these foods is basically never helpful, and many people will have few options beyond them. Intuitive eating will help your client gain awareness of how different foods make them feel physically, without all the shame. It's also worth noting many foods deemed "healthy," including protein bars and shakes and meat substitutes are actually highly processed.

separate category is debatable. If it seems helpful for your client to use the label "play foods," awesome. But if not, let's just call it food. A separate **Rethinking Terminology** handout is available for your reference.

EXERCISE: Rethinking Terminology

1. **Think about the words we use to describe food. For instance, let's think about foods generally considered less nutritious. What are words typically used to describe these foods?**

    The most obvious example is "junk food." Food may also be described as "indulgent," "sinful," or a "guilty pleasure."

2. **Let's think about what those words actually mean. For instance, what comes to mind when you think of "junk"? What about "sinful" or "guilty"?**

    "Junk" is typically used to refer to something without value. "Sinful" and "guilty" imply that one has done something morally wrong. The word "indulgent" suggests something that is excessive and even without control.

3. **Now let's think about the words used to describe foods considered highly nutritious. For instance, how often do you hear foods described as "clean"? What does this suggest?**

    "Clean" implies something is pure; anything not considered "clean" could thus be considered dirty or impure. The words assigned to foods often connote morality and superiority, and they can have enormous power. One may feel superior for eating "good" foods and feel guilty or ashamed for eating "bad" foods.

4. **How could labeling foods as "junk" or "indulgent" contribute to your emotions around eating?**

    At this step, you want to guide your client to consider whether they want a label for these foods at all. As noted, "play food" is certainly an option. But you may also want to consider if these categories potentially continue to perpetuate the good food/bad food dichotomy. For lack of better terminology, I often opt for "nutrient-dense" when describing foods culturally ascribed as "healthy." But even that term is quite vague, given that "nutritious" foods vary greatly in the type and density of macro- and micronutrients present. There's no right answer: the goal is that you get your client thinking about the power of language in shaping our emotions and behaviors!

Step 4: Am I Ready for Gentle Nutrition?

As noted in the intro to this chapter, if your client is still working through making peace with food, you may want to start the session here. Sometimes folks are eager to jump to gentle nutrition, but the motivations for this can get entangled with diet culture. The purpose of this exercise is to help your client explore how much their desire for integrating nutrition into their food choices is coming from a genuine interest in their well-being and not from the remnants of diet culture's rules. It doesn't have to be all or none. Because diet culture surrounds us, it's challenging (if not impossible) to shut it out completely. Instead, you want to explore your client's *primary* motivations AND whether they have the tools to notice and address any diet mentality when it seeps in.

EXERCISE: Am I Ready for Gentle Nutrition?

This exercise works particularly well in a group but is also appropriate for individual sessions. First, you will ask your client or group to brainstorm questions they can ask themselves to help figure out if they are ready to incorporate gentle nutrition. I recommend writing these out on a whiteboard or paper; ideally it would be something your client could reference later.

1. **What are some questions you might ask yourself to figure out if you're ready for gentle nutrition?**

    Allow your client or group to come up with ideas first. Below are some additional questions you might add:

    - Do I still pick foods because I feel like I "should"? Where does the "should" come from?
    - Am I being influenced by people I follow on social media more than by my own internal experience?
    - How rigid are my food choices?
    - What emotions come up when I eat "play" foods?
    - Do I experience guilt after certain food choices?
    - Do I feel better after eating a meal that has variety, including vegetables? Or am I choosing a salad at lunch because I feel guilty for eating what I really want?

2. Am I choosing this food because I want to feel good or because I feel guilty?

    For further reflection, you can provide the exercise's accompanying handout, **Am I Ready for Gentle Nutrition?**, which helps your client consider which intuitive eating principles they may need to continue working on before diving into gentle nutrition. For instance, if your client still feels guilt when eating certain foods because of their nutritional content, they may need to spend more time on making peace with food. *Or* they may notice that they are still using eating or exercise to cope with challenging emotions, suggesting they may need to spend more time on principle seven.

If your client seems discouraged, remind them that good things take time. Because your client has spent a lifetime building patterns and attitudes around food, eating, and their body, developing a new relationship with these won't happen overnight. Gentle nutrition is there when they're ready for it, but if they attempt to dive in too soon, they risk slipping back into old habits.

Step 5: The Pursuit of Progress over Perfection

Intuitive eating represents a huge paradigm shift for many people. We have spent most of our lives learning totally different information (e.g., weight loss = good, sweet foods = bad) and wiring specific behavioral patterns. Shifting perspectives and changing habits is hard work! Tuning in to your own needs and filtering out all the external chatter, over and over again each day, is exhausting! When your client is stressed, busy, or emotional, they may find themselves sliding back into old thought and behavior patterns simply because they lack the bandwidth to do all the introspection required of change.

Gentle nutrition runs a particularly high risk of acquiring rigidity because of the rampant healthism evident in Westernized cultures. Up until this point, your client has been paying attention to other things: their hunger, their food rules, their fullness, their emotions, body image, and movement. After years of being fed messages about "healthy" eating, they got a break from all that. Reintroducing nutrition may be relieving, stressful, or both. Our culture has already given us many heuristics about nutrition. Sugar is bad, protein is good. Processed foods are poison, but produce is medicine (unless you're on the carnivore diet). Therefore, your client may have a hard time compartmentalizing their *own* experiences from these pervasive messages. Because we already have a blueprint to shame ourselves about our food choices, they're more likely to be hard on themselves for eating foods that don't feel good in their body, than for, say, having a negative body-image day.

Therefore, you want to encourage your client to have a curious, growth-oriented mindset. If they have a week where they eat foods they know don't make them feel good, they haven't been "bad," nor was this a "mistake." Humans learn the most when things don't go according to plan. If everything is seamless, there's nothing to learn.

Below are two activities you can do to help your client cultivate this growth mindset; you can skip them if they're not relevant for your client.

EXERCISE: Part 1—How Does Shame Serve Me?

In this first exercise, you will encourage your client to explore the longer-term implications of shame, considering whether self-criticism is helping them eat in alignment with their needs. You can use the **Patience and Progress** handout to guide these exercises (or give them to your client to do between sessions if you run out of time).

> *Think back to a time where you were hard on yourself about your eating. Perhaps you noticed you had fallen into a pattern of eating that wasn't honoring your health, or maybe you ate something you knew wouldn't sit well.*
>
> 1. **How did you talk to yourself? What are examples of the thoughts you had?**
>
> 2. **How did those thoughts make you feel? What emotions came up?**
>
> 3. **How useful were these thoughts? Did they motivate you to make changes or do something differently next time?**

4. If so, were you able to maintain those changes?

5. If self-criticism didn't motivate behavior change, what happened instead?

Now imagine if you viewed the experience with openness and curiosity and did not get hooked by self-criticism. That is, you recognized that the experience provided useful information you could use in the future.

1. **What is it like to imagine taking that approach?**

2. **How do you think being open and curious would affect your motivation to do something differently in the future or make changes?**

3. **What about your emotions? How do you think you'd feel if you viewed that experience as giving you useful information instead of criticizing yourself?**

It's important to remember that self-critical thoughts are likely to come up. The goal is not necessarily to eliminate them (which may not be realistic and could garner even more self-criticism), but rather to not get hooked by them. When we get hooked by self-criticism, it has a powerful effect on our emotions and behaviors. If your client continues to practice greeting these experiences with openness and curiosity, over time they'll get better at noticing the thoughts and letting them pass. Eventually, they may notice the thoughts also pop up less frequently and are less powerful than before.

EXERCISE: Part 2—Practicing Self-Compassion and Curiosity

Now that your client has considered the potential utility or benefits of taking a more self-compassionate and curious approach, it's time to practice what that might look like!

Now that you've considered whether shame is serving you, and reflected on the potential benefits of self-compassion and curiosity, it's time to put these concepts into practice. Think back to that same scenario from the first part of this exercise: a time when you made an eating choice that was out of alignment with your needs.

1. **If this happened again, how might you react to or deal with self-critical thoughts as they come up?**

    The cognitive reframing and defusion skills your client practiced in Session 4 will come in handy here. First, you want your client to notice their thoughts so they can be intentional about how they react. They might be prepared immediately to reframe them. However, the awareness and initiative it takes to notice and reframe thoughts generally come with practice and time and happen under optimal conditions (e.g., not super stressed). Sometimes, your client may not have the bandwidth to engage in cognitive reframing. In those instances, their best course of action may simply be to let the thought pass by. Ultimately, the goal is for your client to reduce how much power their thoughts have over their emotions and behaviors.

Sometimes cognitive reframing is great for that, but letting thoughts pass without getting hooked (i.e., cognitive defusion) can be equally effective.

2. **Thinking of the self-critical thoughts you had about this situation, what are other more balanced and compassionate ways of viewing it?**

    Using the example of the scenario of being lactose-intolerant and eating ice cream, your client may consider:

    Rather than: "I'm bad/weak for eating ice cream."

    Try: "Ice cream is delicious. It makes sense that I wanted to eat some."

    Or: "All my friends were eating ice cream and it looked delicious. Of course I wanted to join them."

    Rather than: "I always do this. I never learn. I'm hopeless."

    Try: "I'm noticing I wasn't very intentional with this decision. I ate ice cream without thinking through how I might feel later. I'm feeling uncomfortable now, but this feeling will pass."

3. **What insights can you gain from this past situation?**

    We will all sometimes eat in ways that aren't aligned with our needs. That's part of being human! In fact, in some situations, it's culturally normative (e.g., holidays). However, if your client is noting consistent patterns that have negative effects, it's worth getting curious about what may be contributing and how they can change these patterns. For instance, maybe your client notices that they eat mindlessly when they get home from work and often feel sick before going to bed. What else could be going on? Are they eating enough during the day? Do they eat with distractions? Is eating helping to meet emotional needs?

4. **How could you integrate this newfound understanding into your future choices without being harsh on yourself?**

    Let's take the example of eating dairy when you're lactose-intolerant. As I mentioned in the last chapter, I love queso dip, but queso dip doesn't always love me. It would be easy to overgeneralize and decide I can't *ever* have queso because sometimes I experience GI distress after eating it. But that's not the only option! For this situation, I've decided that what works for me is to be more intentional about eating queso. I now ask myself: how is eating queso right now likely to make me feel? Am I OK with feeling that way? Are there ways that I can reduce the likelihood of feeling uncomfortable after eating it? Sometimes I decide it's not worth it to eat queso; maybe I have an event to attend later and don't want to risk GI upset. However, with curiosity and self-compassion, I've been able to learn that I can tolerate queso when I eat a smaller portion and am mindful about what foods I pair with it (e.g., less dairy).

    The point is: you want to encourage your client's flexibility. In some instances, your client may need to avoid foods or situations altogether. Food allergies are obvious, but your client may decide that the effects they get from eating beans, for instance, simply aren't worth it (especially if they don't love beans). It's easy to get rigid with our nutrition and sometimes this rigidity can be diet culture–driven (e.g., someone may jump at the possibility of swearing off French fries). So you want to guide your client toward choices that are right for them—which will look different for everyone—*not* what diet culture says is right.

OPTIONAL EXERCISE: What Is Food For?

Spending a lifetime bombarded by often conflicting messages about health, food, bodies, weight, and appearance can lead us to forget the purposes of food and why we even eat it in the first place! Some of your clients may be so focused on eating the "right" things that they forget to check in on how those "right" foods even make them feel. Others may be so concerned with how what they eat will affect their shape and/or weight that they aren't thinking about what foods actually do in the body. Still others may be focused primarily on how foods *taste* or meet emotional needs, such that they're not thinking much about how foods make them feel or how they promote their well-being. More than likely, it's a mix of all the above.

The **What Is Food For?** exercise is designed to get your client thinking about the purpose of food, and what it actually does for us. If your client has struggled with viewing foods as good or bad, still has the tendency to get rigid about "clean" eating or assign morality to foods, or has difficulty moving away from self-criticism and shame, you may want to skip this exercise. The last thing we want is for this exercise to make your client feel bad about how they view food or to encourage any sort of healthism; for example, believing food's *only* purpose is to meet nutritional needs.

Start with a simple question: Why do we eat? Or, what is the purpose of eating and food? With your client, jot down a list. Some potential options are:

- Energy
- Muscle function
- Growth
- Repair of injuries or illness
- Celebration
- Connection
- Joy
- Stamina

- Disease prevention
- Keeps the organs running
- Insulation for the brain
- Insulation for the joints
- To build muscles
- To move the body
- To participate in life
- To boost mood

You can get more granular, noting physiological functions like eyesight, cardiovascular function, brain function, and more. For instance, vitamin C and zinc are well known for their connection to the immune system. Carrots are chock-full of vitamin A, which is instrumental for vision, among other things. You can get potassium from bananas and leafy greens, and it is a key mineral that assists in maintaining blood pressure, water balance, muscle contractions, and heart rhythm. Many people dismiss carbohydrates, but they provide energy and help regulate insulin.

It's also important to acknowledge nonphysiological benefits of food and eating. Food is a way we connect with others, celebrate holidays and achievements, and experience pleasure and joy. We don't want to become so focused on how foods serve our physical health that we lose sight of how they affect our well-being more broadly.

Now, ask your client to pick three to five food purposes that really resonate with them, to use as affirmations. For instance: "Food is connection;" "Food is *not* punishment;" and "This meal gives me energy and boosts my mood." The goal is that, if your client is ever losing sight of the bigger picture, they have a few affirmations handy to help shift their perspective. Your client may choose to save these in a note on their phone, set an alarm for them to pop up at mealtimes, add them to a phone wallpaper, or even post sticky notes on their mirror. Encourage them to get creative and experiment with what will be most helpful.

Step 6: Between-Session Exercises and Closing

The between-session exercises this week will depend on your client's readiness to approach gentle nutrition. If your client feels ready to begin exploring how different foods make them feel in the short and long term, they'll practice the **Body–Food Choice Congruence** exercise two or three times this week. Encourage your client to plan ahead, choosing to reflect on meals or snacks that happen when they have a little extra time to jot down notes before and after eating. The exercise will be similar to what you practiced in session. Before eating, your client will check in with themselves about whether they are experiencing any cravings or preferences for certain foods. Are they able to identify foods that not only sound good taste-wise, but also will make them feel good? For instance, let's say your client starts work early and doesn't get a break for six hours. What foods could they choose to eat before work that they enjoy and that will give them enough energy to last until their break? To answer this question, it's useful to think about how potential food options have made their body feel in the past. Maybe your client is choosing between eggs, toast, and fruit, or a bowl of cereal with a banana. Which meal gave them the sustained energy they needed to get through the shift? How did the foods feel in their body? What would feel best today?

After the meal or snack, your client will briefly check in on how it went. It can be especially helpful for your client to do this at their *next* meal or snack, as they'll have more time to judge how the eating experience went. How did the foods feel in their body? Did they experience fullness *and* satisfaction? What was the quality of the fullness sensation (e.g., unpleasant, neutral, pleasant)? Did they learn anything from that particular meal or snack?

I want to reiterate: This is intended as a useful practice that can help your client be intentional with their food choices. Over time, this practice should become more automatic and less cognitively effortful. The goal is *not* to encourage overthinking. If your client is feeling overwhelmed practicing body–food choice congruence, they can scale it back. This might look like doing the exercise just one or two times a week, or generating two or three questions your client can ask themselves after a meal to quickly gauge how it made their body feel.

If your client is struggling with impatience or feeling self-critical about their progress, encourage them to do the **Patience and Progress** exercise on their own this week, ideally at least twice. Finally, if your client isn't quite ready for gentle nutrition, spend a little time assessing which principles they may need to revisit. For instance, if they're still struggling to let go of dieting because they're holding onto hope of changing their body, you may want to repeat some exercises from Session 7 (Body Respect) and potentially Session 1 (Ditching Dieting).

Closing

As always, mutually share what will stick with you and your client or group members from this session.

Session 9: Gentle Nutrition

Lengthening the Session

If time and resources permit, this session can be expanded into two. Lengthening this session would be most beneficial for clients who are:

- Ready for gentle nutrition
- Still dealing with self-criticism around their food choices
- Returning to gentle nutrition after revisiting other principles
- Experiencing difficulty identifying how foods feel in their bodies
- Struggling to differentiate cravings from body–food choice congruence

To lengthen this session, I suggest:

- Spending the first session on Steps 1, 2, and 3
- Spending the second session on Steps 4 and 5

Shortening the Session

You may be able to shorten or skip this session if you and/or your client know they're not ready for gentle nutrition quite yet. To shorten the session, briefly introduce body–food choice congruence (Step 2), but skip the exercise and move straight to Step 4 (Am I Ready for Gentle Nutrition?). If you have time, you can discuss the power of our language in shaping how we feel about food (Step 3) and/or do the self-compassion exercises in Step 5, depending on your client's needs.

CHAPTER 13

Session 10: Celebrating Progress and Planning for the Future

Session Outline

Step 1: Between-Session Exercises Debriefing

  Body–Food Choice Congruence

  Patience and Progress

Step 2: Celebrating Progress

  Handout: Growing as an Intuitive Eater Plan

  Exercise: Reflecting on Progress

Step 3: Looking Ahead

  Exercise: Planning for the Future

Step 4: Benefits and Closing

  Exercise: Reflecting on the Program

  Sample Growing as an Intuitive Eater Plan

Materials

Growing as an Intuitive Eater

Session Aim

You've made it! To get to this point, you and your client have put in an immense amount of work. Your client has begun to dismantle the harmful beliefs they've absorbed about food and bodies; is learning how to notice, trust, and honor their body's needs; and is working to respect and appreciate their body, find joy in movement, and maybe even consider how foods feel in their body.

This is an exciting point, but also a scary point. Whenever I wrap up an intuitive eating intervention with a client, I feel a mix of emotions: inspiration and pride for how far they've come, excitement for how intuitive eating will positively shape their life, and fear of their returning to a world saturated with misinformation and weight obsession with less structure and support. Therefore, the purpose of this session is to take inventory of how far your client has come: how their perspectives and behaviors have shifted, and how these shifts have impacted their lives broadly. You want to help your client see and celebrate their progress. It's also important to consider how your client can keep their progress going and how they can navigate triggers and threats to their newfound perspective. Despite all the progress they may have made, they're just getting started! It takes time to ingrain beliefs and behaviors, and your client will be more vulnerable initially to triggers in their environment. Therefore, you want to help your client think ahead to how they can protect themselves and cope when challenging situations arise.

To structure this session, you'll be creating a **Growing as an Intuitive Eater Plan** that encapsulates progress and charts a plan for the future. There is a blueprint of this exercise included at the end of this chapter, but modify as needed, including changing the title to suit your client. The goal is that your client walks out of this last session feeling proud and empowered to move forward.

Additional Considerations and Potential Adaptations

If your client isn't quite ready to wrap up yet, or you perceive they need a bit more time, refer to the Appendix for considerations on how to move forward.

> ## Considerations for Group Interventions
>
> This session is especially powerful in a group format. Participants get to celebrate and reflect together, be validated for any difficult emotions that arise (e.g., disappointment, fear), and brainstorm ways to keep the momentum going. However, as always, social comparison is likely. Some participants may seem especially confident about their progress, or seem to have made greater leaps than most. Others may be feeling insecure, fearful, or disappointed that they haven't made as much progress as they hoped. Some are going to have an easier path forward, like those who hold multiple privileged identities. Throughout the session, be sure to validate the range of experiences and emotions people have. Everyone has different starting lines and life circumstances that make direct comparisons unfair.
>
> Encourage group members who are interested to keep in touch. Connecting with the other members is a way to build an accepting and supportive community, which makes intuitive eating easier *and* more sustainable.

Step 1: Between-Session Exercises Debriefing

Your client had a few options for between-session exercises. If they were ready to tackle gentle nutrition, they may have practiced the **Body–Food Choice Congruence** exercise two to three times. Do they have any global observations from the exercise? For instance, how easy was it to identify foods that would be satisfying and feel good in their bodies? Did they notice any patterns regarding how different foods made them feel, such as energy level, concentration, staying power, or mood? How was their self-talk? Did they notice any adjustments they may want to make in the future?

If your client engages in frequent self-criticism, you may have asked them to practice self-compassion and curiosity with the **Patience and Progress** activity. How many times did they practice over the week? What types of self-critical thoughts came up? How did they respond? Were they able to defuse from the thoughts and take an open, curious stance? What was it like to move from self-criticism to self-compassion?

Step 2: Celebrating Progress

Refer to the **Growing as an Intuitive Eater Plan** handout to guide the remainder of the session. There's an example plan at the end of this chapter to demonstrate what one might look like.

EXERCISE: Reflecting on Progress

In this step, you'll help your client reflect on how they've grown and what they've learned. Doing so helps to encapsulate their progress and prepare them for the road ahead. Throughout this exercise, encourage your client to get specific!

1. **What was my "why"?**

    First, you and your client will revisit their original goals. What did they want out of this experience? What did they hope would change? Try to be as concrete as possible; hopefully you and your client have been revisiting these goals throughout the intervention.

2. **Where am I now?**

    Where is your client now in relation to their original goals? Validate and celebrate any progress: they have spent decades forming their relationships with their body and with food. Lasting change doesn't happen overnight. Perhaps your client still experiences discomfort when their partner touches them, or feels a sense of dread imagining shopping for clothes. Are they engaging in more values-committed actions (e.g., feeling their fear and doing a valued action anyway)? Or perhaps your client used to think of their body only in terms of its shape or size, but are now beginning to appreciate some of the amazing things their body does, like recovering from illness.

    Also allow space for your client to process and move through any disappointment or grief. Perhaps your client hoped this process would be easier, or they'd be farther along. If they haven't made as much progress as they hoped, what stories are they are telling themselves about why this is so? Be on the lookout for undue self-criticism or shame. Any barriers your client is experiencing to progress are rich data to integrate moving forward. Check out the Appendix for ideas about how to move forward if your client seems stuck.

    Ideally, you can write out several concrete examples of steps your client has made throughout your time together. I find that folks often struggle to give themselves credit, so if your client minimizes their growth, share the progress you've seen. Having tangible examples of progress can keep your client motivated and moving forward.

3. **What have I learned? What has helped me so far?**

    Explore with your client what they've learned about themselves—and even about the world! Have some of their beliefs about food and body image changed? What insights have they had about their own needs and priorities? For instance, maybe they realized that following strict diet rules isn't keeping them safe or helping them achieve their life goals. Or maybe they realized they benefit from structure around their eating, such as eating every three to four hours or engaging in meal planning once a week.

    Understanding what has helped your client make progress is important data for how to keep that progress going. Refer back to the areas of progress they noted with the last question. What specific factors helped them get there? Are there supportive people in their life who they can confide in? Did they set boundaries in relationships or improve communication? Donate clothes that no longer fit? Change their social media habits?

Step 3: Looking Ahead

Hopefully, the last exercise helped your client acknowledge and internalize their progress, which should increase their self-efficacy. Nevertheless, your client likely still has areas where they'd like to grow and goals they want to achieve.

EXERCISE: Planning for the Future

This step is designed to help your client set goals, consider what they'll need to achieve them, and walk through how they'll protect their progress and respond to challenges. As with the last exercise, it's best if your client gets specific about their goals. They may have overarching goals, like developing body appreciation or decreasing their emotional eating. However, such goals are usually pretty broad and can feel daunting and abstract on their own. Getting specific will help your client break these goals down into tangible steps.

1. **What is my "why" now?**

   What are your client's reasons for continuing to move forward? On the **Growing as an Intuitive Eater Plan**, you'll notice there is space for your client to elaborate on their "why" for all ten intuitive eating principles. For instance, there's space for them to explore why it's important that they keep challenging their food rules and engaging in mindful movement. You likely won't have time in session to discuss all of these, so at minimum, discuss their overall reasons for moving forward.

2. **What are my goals moving forward?**

   What concrete goals does your client have now around food, movement, and body image? It's OK if they want to stay the course with their previous goals, but this is a great opportunity for them to revisit and revise. If they project five, ten, even fifteen years into the future, what do they want their relationship with their body, food, and movement to look like? It's OK if your client has a broad, overarching goal like improving their body image; yet, without breaking that goal down into smaller steps, it's likely to feel daunting and hard to get started. What steps can they take to get there?

3. **What would help me achieve these goals?**

   What does your client need to achieve their goals? Likely, they can draw from some of the things that have helped them so far. Some ideas could be finding affirming, weight-inclusive medical providers; building or strengthening their social network and community (e.g., joining a hiking club or taking pottery classes); being mindful of social media use; engaging in valued activities (e.g., reading, art, volunteering). What's accessible to your client will vary, but the more your client is able to participate fully in life, the less room there is for poor body image or disordered eating.

4. **What could get in the way?**

   Being aware of triggers and roadblocks that could derail progress is crucial to prepare your client to navigate these situations as they arise. When you spot a bump in the road, you're able to slow your speed and get through the obstacle safely. Without preparation, you're more likely to be thrown off course. If your client struggles to think of examples, ask them what situations have been triggering or resulted in increased struggles with food and body image in the past. There are many possibilities, including holidays, body-related changes, relationship difficulties (e.g., breakups), grief, traumatic events, social media, and more.

5. **How will I know if I'm slipping back into old patterns?**

   Explore the signs your client may be slipping back into old thought or behavior patterns. For instance, are they becoming more socially withdrawn? Having more distressing body-related thoughts? Avoiding certain situations or activities due to concerns about body image and/or food? Feeling enticed to try new diets or nutrition tips they heard about on social media or through family/friends?

6. **What can I do when I notice I am struggling?**

   If your client notices signs they are returning to old thought patterns/behaviors, what are ways they can respond? As always, be as specific as possible! Think of it as a kind of safety plan—what are five discrete steps they could take? Refer to the completed **Growing as an Intuitive Eater Plan** at the end of the chapter for an example of how this might look.

7. **How can I stay vigilant against diet culture?**

   This last question is crucial. Weight stigma is pervasive and intersects with many other forms of oppression. We are bombarded with often conflicting, over-hyped, and even inaccurate information about nutrition and health. It's impossible to avoid. Further, it can be insidious. Your client might hear a podcast with a neuroscientist proclaiming the keto diet will solve the mental health crisis and feel curious. After all, who doesn't want to improve their mental health? As we are increasingly saturated by information, it's hard to parse through what is true and unbiased. Even when there's evidence eating a certain way can improve a health marker, it doesn't mean that way of eating is right for *your* client. Diet culture is pervasive and powerful and may slowly pull your client back in. What are ways they can remain vigilant without being *hyper*vigilant?

   One important note: if your client is genuinely curious whether changing their eating patterns could benefit their health, it's important they talk to a professional. A dietitian trained in eating disorders, for instance, could help them determine whether making changes would ultimately be beneficial or harmful and then guide them toward making any changes safely.

Step 4: Benefits and Closing

EXERCISE: Reflecting on the Program

At the end of this session, you can wrap up by asking your client any of the following questions. I find this exercise works especially well in a group setting, as it helps to strengthen the bonds members have formed. Some of these questions may feel redundant with Step 2, however they are meant to assess satisfaction with the intervention itself. You can modify or skip any that seem less relevant or extraneous.

1. **What have you taken away from this program?**

2. **How has this experience changed your beliefs around food, body image, and exercise?**

3. **How has this experience changed the way you approach coping with difficult emotions?**

4. **How has this experience changed the way you feel about your body?**

5. **How are you feeling about your ability to continue working on your relationship with food, body image, and exercise moving forward?**

After this reflection, close out by sharing what this experience has meant for you. Be authentic! In piloting this intervention, it was clear to us that participants benefited from and appreciated our vulnerability. Any self-disclosures should of course be appropriate and for the benefit of your clients, but touching on how you have also grown and learned from your client can contribute to their healing.

Finally, if you're ending your work with your client or group, be sure to have a list of resources available for them. These can include contact information for local or virtual providers, book and article recommendations, social media accounts to follow, and more. I encourage you to compile your own list, but some of my favorite resources are included in the free tools found at http://www.newharbinger.com/52540.

Great work! You've made it! In the Appendix, I share considerations for when your client may need extra time. The online tools also have some case examples of what intuitive eating can look like with different clients.

SAMPLE GROWING AS AN INTUITIVE EATER PLAN

Progress & Reasons for Change

Since starting this intervention, I'm most proud of:

Confronting fears! I've taken so many steps I never thought I'd be able to take. I'm learning that the more I face my fears, the less power they have over me.

The changes I have made that help me be a more intuitive eater include:

I unfollowed and muted a lot of people on social media. I committed to stopping talking to my partner and my friends about my weight and eating. I've been trying new coping strategies. I'm moving my body in ways that feel good instead of just hard. I'm getting better at identifying when I'm hungry and full.

The most important things that I have learned include:

The more I face the things I'm afraid of, the easier it gets. I have to be really mindful of how I use social media. My hunger and fullness signals actually have a purpose!

It's important for me to continue…

Making peace with food and challenging food rules because:

I want to keep showing up for my partner, my family, and my friends. I'm less present when I'm obsessing about my body and food.

Honoring my hunger and fullness because:

I actually feel better when I'm listening to my body. I'm not getting exhausted in the middle of the day nor am I bingeing at night and waking up with reflux.

Coping with emotions without using food/exercise behaviors because:

This one is really hard, but I do think the more I take care of my body and try new ways to cope, the more stable I feel emotionally. The ways I used to cope weren't helping me in the long run.

Respecting and accepting my body because:

I am starting to believe that my body is more than how it looks. I appreciate my body more now. I don't always like how it looks. But it's just a relief to not have to keep fighting it.

Engaging in mindful movement and gentle nutrition because:

Again, I feel better! I was so tired before. I was using exercise as punishment—to make up for eating. I was often bingeing on foods that didn't make me feel good because I was under-eating during the day. I have to keep working on it because I don't ever want to feel again how I used to feel.

Maintenance of Changes

Ways I can keep working on…

Making peace with food/challenging food rules:

Continue working on my feared food hierarchy; do exposures 1–2x week. Practice thought reframing when unhelpful thoughts pop up. Reach out to my friend for meal support when I'm struggling.

Honoring my hunger/fullness:

Continue practicing eating without screens at least twice/week (usually dinners Tuesday/Friday). Don't overthink hunger—just eat when you're hungry and observe after how your body feels.

Coping with my emotions without using behaviors:

Cope ahead! On Sunday, journal what's coming up and what might trigger urges. Plan for how I'll respond to any challenges. Reach out to loved ones and be honest about how I'm feeling. Continue eating 3 meals and 2–3 snacks/day so I know I'm not irritable due to hunger.

Respecting and accepting my body:

Give away my scale. I've already unfollowed most of the social media accounts that were triggering, but need to stay vigilant there. Give away old clothes that don't fit, and buy clothes that fit my body now. Keep up the writing exercises—those are helpful!

Mindful movement and gentle nutrition:

When meal planning for the week, take into account how the foods typically sit and how much staying power they have. Modify according to my schedule. Continue going to exercise classes with Becky at the Y—I really enjoy those and they don't feel punishing. Going to try skiing this year for the first time—not as punishment but as a new, fun experience. It'll be good for me to be a beginner at something.

Preparation and Prevention

It is important to stay aware of things that will make it difficult to continue working on intuitive eating. Signs that I might be slipping back into my old patterns include:

Pinning recipes (food obsession). Researching diets. Buying another scale. Talking about my body more to others. Getting rigid in my food choices. Feeling guilt around eating. Avoiding intimacy with my partner.

Things I can do to prepare for and respond to these challenges include:

Tell my partner what's going on as soon as I notice it and ask for specific ways he can support me (e.g., eating meals with me, going grocery shopping instead of me). Take a social media break. Take a week off of more intense movement and instead go for walks and do light yoga.

Appendix

What If My Client Needs More Time?

After covering the ten principles, you may feel like your client needs more time. If resources permit, by all means extend the intervention! At this point, you likely have a sense of which principles are difficult for your client. They may need more practice noticing their hunger, more time challenging their food-related rules, more body image–focused work, or more time with gentle nutrition. However, it's important to always consider your client's context.

Consider the following questions:

1. **Are there changes that could be made outside of your sessions to further foster your client's growth?** If your client has insurance coverage, time, and financial resources, working with both a dietitian and a therapist will likely be beneficial—especially when care is collaborative and coordinated. If not, are there free or low-cost online or local resources that might help your client? For instance, many eating disorder–trained dietitians offer online support groups with sliding scale or scholarship options. Or, are you able to get consultation to support your client's lingering concerns?

2. **Does your client need connections to other services, such as psychiatric care, food assistance, housing support, or other health care?** It will be extremely challenging for your client to focus on their body image or eating concerns if they are experiencing such serious issues as poverty, food insecurity, or health concerns.

3. **Are there ways to expand your client's social support or build their community?** This could mean connecting your client to eating- and body image–specific organizations/groups, such as the FEDUP Collective (a collective of trans+, intersex, and gender-diverse people focused on community healing and eating disorder advocacy) or the ANAD Recovery Mentorship Program. However, it may also mean helping your client connect with people with mutual interests or hobbies or encouraging them to become more involved in their spiritual community. It may also mean getting more involved in volunteering or advocacy. Indeed, community-building and advocacy can be important components of healing (Chioneso et al., 2020; French et al., 2020).

4. **Is intuitive eating not the right approach (at least right now)?** It is possible your client isn't responding to intuitive eating. There are many potential reasons for this. If your client's eating or body image concerns are severe or have worsened, they may require more intensive or focused eating disorder treatment. It's critical you assess your client's

progress and symptoms regularly to evaluate whether a higher level of care or different modality is needed. It's also possible intuitive eating may need modification for your client. For instance, we lack data on how to adapt intuitive eating to meet the needs of neurodivergent people, people with chronic health conditions, and those with ARFID. If your client isn't making progress or doesn't feel intuitive eating is working for them, don't force it! Speak with your client to understand their needs and collaborate to find the best approach. It's also possible to integrate intuitive eating principles into other approaches. For instance, many of the goals of enhanced cognitive behavioral therapy (CBT-E) align with intuitive eating principles, including normalizing eating patterns and avoiding dieting. Because intuitive eating promotes interoceptive awareness, it also complements acceptance and commitment therapy and mindfulness-based practices. Finally, you may need additional training in intuitive eating or to refer your client to a certified intuitive eating counselor.

5. **Are there co-occurring diagnoses or other concerns that should be addressed first?**
It is possible your client has other concerns that need support before focusing on eating and body image. For instance, other mental health concerns like posttraumatic stress disorder, substance use disorder, or obsessive-compulsive disorder may need treatment first. Additionally, if your client is experiencing disproportionate inequities or discrimination, they will likely benefit from support that specifically addresses those stressors and trauma. If you do not have the relevant expertise or skills to address the issues your client is facing, a referral may be necessary. If a referral is not possible (due to lack of local providers or insurance coverage, for example), then your seeking training and consultation will help you meet the needs of your client and avoid iatrogenic harm.

References

Academy for Eating Disorders. (2020). *A guide to selecting evidence-based psychological therapies for eating disorders.* https://www.nceedus.org/wp-content/uploads/2022/04/FINAL_AED_Psychological_book.pdf.

Ackard, D. M., Fulkerson, J. A., & Neumark-Sztainer, D. R. (2011). Stability of eating disorder diagnostic classifications in adolescents: Five-year longitudinal findings from a population-based study. *Eating Disorders, 19*(4), 308–322. https://doi.org/10.1080/10640266.2011.584804.

Alleva, J. M., Martijn, C., Van Breukelen, G. J. P., Jansen, A., & Karos, K. (2015). Expand your horizon: A programme that improves body image and reduces self-objectification by training women to focus on body functionality. *Body Image, 15*, 81–89. https://doi.org/10.1016/j.bodyim.2015.07.001.

Almazan, A. N., & Keuroghlian, A. S. (2021). Association between gender-affirming surgeries and mental health outcomes. *JAMA Surgery, 156*(7), 611–618. https://doi.org/10.1001/jamasurg.2021.0952.

Andersen, A. E., & Hay, A. (1985). Racial and socioeconomic: Influences in anorexia nervosa and bulimia. *International Journal of Eating Disorders, 4*(4), 479–487. https://doi.org/10.1002/1098-108X(198511)4:4%3C479::AID-EAT2260040408%3E3.0.CO;2-R.

Andrew, R., Tiggemann, M., & Clark, L. (2014). An extension of the acceptance model of intuitive eating in adolescent girls: A role for social comparison? *Journal of Eating Disorders, 2*(Suppl 1), O40. https://doi.org/10.1186/2050-2974-2-S1-O40.

Augustus-Horvath, C. L., & Tylka, T. L. (2011). The acceptance model of intuitive eating: A comparison of women in emerging adulthood, early adulthood, and middle adulthood. *Journal of Counseling Psychology, 58*(1), 110–125. https://doi.org/10.1037/a0022129.

Avalos, L. C., & Tylka, T. L. (2006). Exploring a model of intuitive eating with college women. *Journal of Counseling Psychology, 53*(4), 486–497. https://doi.org/10.1037/0022-0167.53.4.486.

Bacon, L., Aphramor, L., Kuller, L., Savage, M., Hirsch, I., Siegler, I., et al. (2011). Weight science: Evaluating the evidence for a paradigm shift. *Nutrition Journal, 10*(1), 9. https://doi.org/10.1186/1475-2891-10-9.

Bacon, L., Stern, J. S., Van Loan, M. D., & Keim, N. L. (2005). Size acceptance and intuitive eating improve health for obese, female chronic dieters. *Journal of the American Dietetic Association, 105*(6), 929–936. https://doi.org/10.1016/j.jada.2005.03.011.

Barad, A., Cartledge, A., Gemmill, K., Misner, N. M., Santiago, C. E., Yavelow, M., & Langkamp-Henken, B. (2019). Associations between intuitive eating behaviors and fruit and vegetable intake among college students. *Journal of Nutrition Education and Behavior, 51*(6), 758–762. https://doi.org/10.1016/j.jneb.2019.03.010.

Becker, C. B., & Stice, E. (2017). From efficacy to effectiveness to broad implementation: Evolution of the Body Project. *Journal of Consulting and Clinical Psychology, 85*(8), 767–782. https://doi.org/10.1037/ccp0000204.

Belon, K. E., Serier, K. N., VanderJagt, H., & Smith, J. E. (2022). What is healthy eating? Exploring profiles of intuitive eating and nutritionally healthy eating in college women. *American Journal of Health Promotion, 36*(5), 823–833. https://doi.org/10.1177/08901171211073870.

Bhattacharya, A., Cooper, M., McAdams, C., Peebles, R., & Timko, C. A. (2022). Cultural shifts in the symptoms of Anorexia Nervosa: The case of Orthorexia Nervosa. *Appetite, 170*, 105869. https://doi.org/10.1016/j.appet.2021.105869.

Black, M. J., Sokol, N., & Vartanian, L. R. (2014). The effect of effort and weight controllability on perceptions of obese individuals. *Journal of Social Psychology, 154*(6), 515–526. https://doi.org/10.1080/00224545.2014.953025.

Braun, T. D., Park, C. L., & Gorin, A. (2016). Self-compassion, body image, and disordered eating: A review of the literature. *Body Image, 17*, 117–131. https://doi.org/10.1016/j.bodyim.2016.03.003.

Brehm, J. W. (1966). *A theory of psychological reactance.* New York: Academic Press.

Brooks, S., & Severson, A. (2022). *How to raise an intuitive eater: Raising the next generation with food and body confidence.* New York: St. Martin's Essentials.

Brown, T. A., & Lavender, J. M. (2021). Eating disorders and body image across the lifespan: A focus on boys and men in midlife and beyond. In J. M. Nagata, T. A. Brown, S. B. Murray, & J. M Lavender (Eds.), *Eating disorders in boys and men* (pp. 317–333). Cham, Switzerland: Springer Nature. https://doi.org/10.1007/978-3-030-67127-3_21.

Brownell, K. D., Kersh, R., Ludwig, D. S., Post, R. C., Puhl, R. M., Schwartz, M. B., & Willett, W. C. (2010). Personal responsibility and obesity: A constructive approach to a controversial issue. *Health Affairs, 29*(3), 379–387. https://doi.org/10.1377/hlthaff.2009.0739.

Burke, N. L., Hazzard, V. M., Schaefer, L. M., Simone, M., O'Flynn, J. L., & Rodgers, R. F. (2023). Socioeconomic status and eating disorder prevalence: At the intersections of gender identity, sexual orientation, and race/ethnicity. *Psychological Medicine, 53*(9), 4255–4265. https://doi.org/10.1017/S0033291722001015.

Burke, N. L., Schaefer, L. M., Hazzard, V. M., & Rodgers, R. F. (2020). Where identities converge: The importance of intersectionality in eating disorders research. *International Journal of Eating Disorders, 53*(10), 1605–1609. https://doi.org/10.1002/eat.23371.

Burlingame, G. M., McClendon, D. T., & Yang, C. (2018). Cohesion in group therapy: A meta-analysis. *Psychotherapy, 55*, 384–398. https://doi.org/10.1037/pst0000173.

Burnette, C. B., Burt, S. A., & Klump, K. L. (2023). The ignored role of disadvantage in eating disorders. *Trends in Molecular Medicine, 30*(4), 305–307. https://doi.org/10.1016/j.molmed.2023.11.006.

Burnette, C. B., Hazzard, V. M., Hahn, S. L., Larson, N., & Neumark-Sztainer, D. (2022). Like parent, like child? Intuitive eating among emerging adults and their parents. *Appetite, 176*, 106132. https://doi.org/10.1016/j.appet.2022.106132.

Burnette, C. B., Hazzard, V. M., Larson, N., Hahn, S. L., Eisenberg, M. E., & Neumark-Sztainer, D. (2023). Is intuitive eating a privileged approach? Cross-sectional and longitudinal associations between food insecurity and intuitive eating. *Public Health Nutrition, 26*(7), 1358–1367. https://doi.org/10.1017/S1368980023000460.

Burnette, C. B., Hazzard, V. M., Linardon, J., Rodgers, R. F., Loth, K. A., & Neumark-Sztainer, D. (2023). How parental feeding practices relate to young people's intuitive eating: Cross-sectional and longitudinal associations by gender and weight concern. *Journal of Adolescent Health, 73*(6), 1145–1152. https://doi.org/10.1016/j.jadohealth.2023.07.018.

Burnette, C. B., Luzier, J. L., Weisenmuller, C. M., & Boutté, R. L. (2022). A systematic review of sociodemographic reporting and representation in eating disorder psychotherapy treatment trials in the United States. *International Journal of Eating Disorders, 55*(4), 423–454. https://doi.org/10.1002/eat.23699.

Burnette, C. B., & Mazzeo, S. E. (2020). An uncontrolled pilot feasibility trial of an intuitive eating intervention for college women with disordered eating delivered through group and guided self-help modalities. *International Journal of Eating Disorders, 53*(9), 1405–1417. https://doi.org/10.1002/eat.23319.

Calzo, J. P., Blashill, A. J., Brown, T. A., & Argenal, R. L. (2017). Eating disorders and disordered weight and shape control behaviors in sexual minority populations. *Current Psychiatry Reports, 19*(8), Article 49. https://doi.org/10.1007/s11920-017-0801-y.

References

Camilleri, G. M., Méjean, C., Bellisle, F., Andreeva, V. A., Kesse-Guyot, E., Hercberg, S., & Péneau, S. (2016). Intuitive eating dimensions were differently associated with food intake in the general population-based NutriNet-Santé study. *The Journal of Nutrition, 147*(1), 61–69. https://doi.org/10.3945/jn.116.234088.

Capodilupo, C. M. (2015). One size does not fit all: Using variables other than the thin ideal to understand Black women's body image. *Cultural Diversity and Ethnic Minority Psychology, 21*(2), 268–278. https://doi.org/10.1037/a0037649.

Capodilupo, C. M., & Kim, S. (2014). Gender and race matter: The importance of considering intersections in Black women's body image. *Journal of Counseling Psychology, 61*(1), 37–49. https://doi.org/10.1037/a0034597.

Castle, M., & Aphramor, L. (2022). The unbearable straightness of intuitive eating. In P. Joy & M. Aston (Eds.), *Queering Nutrition and Dietetics*. New York: Routledge.

Chapman, J., & Woodman, T. (2016). Disordered eating in male athletes: A meta-analysis. *Journal of Sports Sciences, 34*(2), 101–109. https://doi.org/10.1080/02640414.2015.1040824.

Cheng, Z. H., Perko, V. L., Fuller-Marashi, L., Gau, J. M., & Stice, E. (2019). Ethnic differences in eating disorder prevalence, risk factors, and predictive effects of risk factors among young women. *Eating Behaviors, 32*, 23–30. https://doi.org/10.1016/j.eatbeh.2018.11.004.

Cheshire, A., Berry, M., & Fixsen, A. (2020). What are the key features of orthorexia nervosa and influences on its development? A qualitative investigation. *Appetite, 155*, 104798. https://doi.org/10.1016/j.appet.2020.104798.

Chioneso, N. A., Hunter, C. D., Gobin, R. L., McNeil Smith, S., Mendenhall, R., & Neville, H. A. (2020). Community healing and resistance through storytelling: A framework to address racial trauma in Africana communities. *Journal of Black Psychology, 46*(2–3), 95–121. https://doi.org/10.1177/0095798420929468.

Christoph, M. J., Hazzard, V. M., Järvelä-Reijonen, E., Hooper, L., Larson, N., & Neumark-Sztainer, D. R. (2021). Intuitive eating is associated with higher fruit and vegetable intake among adults. *Journal of Nutrition Education and Behavior, 53*(3), 240–245. https://doi.org/10.1016/j.jneb.2020.11.015.

Christoph, M. J., Järvelä-Reijonen, E., Hooper, L., Larson, N., Mason, S. M., & Neumark-Sztainer, D. R. (2021). Longitudinal associations between intuitive eating and weight-related behaviors in a population-based sample of young adults. *Appetite, 160*, 105093. https://doi.org/10.1016/j.appet.2021.105093.

Coleman-Jensen, A., Rabbitt, M. P., Gregory, C. A., & Singh, A. (2021). *Household food security in the United States in 2020*. U.S. Department of Agriculture, Economic Research Service.

Colles, S. L., Dixon, J. B., & O'Brien, P. E. (2008). Loss of control is central to psychological disturbance associated with binge eating disorder. *Obesity, 16*(3), 608–614. https://doi.org/10.1038/oby.2007.99.

Convertino, A. D., Brady, J. P., Albright, C. A., Gonzales, M., & Blashill, A. J. (2021). The role of sexual minority stress and community involvement on disordered eating, dysmorphic concerns and appearance- and performance-enhancing drug misuse. *Body Image, 36*, 53–63. https://doi.org/10.1016/J.bodyim.2020.10.006.

Crimmins, E. M., Hayward, M. D., & Seeman, T. E. (2004). Race/ethnicity, socioeconomic status, and health. In N. B. Anderson, R. A. Bulatao, & B. Cohen (Eds.), *Critical Perspectives on Racial and Ethnic Differences in Health in Late Life* (pp. 310–352). Washington, DC: National Academies Press. https://www.ncbi.nlm.nih.gov/books/NBK25526.

Crowther, J. H., Tennenbaum, D. L., Hobfoll, S. E., & Stephens, M. A. P. (2013). Chronic dieting and eating disorders: A spiral model. *The Etiology of Bulimia Nervosa: The Individual and Familial Context*, 149–172. https://doi.org/10.4324/9780203782286-15.

Dakanalis, A., Colmegna, F., Riva, G., & Clerici, M. (2017). Validity and utility of the DSM-5 severity specifier for binge-eating disorder. *International Journal of Eating Disorders, 50*(8), 917–923. https://doi.org/10.1002/eat.22696.

Davies, A. E., Burnette, C. B., Ravyts, S. G., & Mazzeo, S. E. (2022). A randomized control trial of Expand Your Horizon: An intervention for women with weight bias internalization. *Body Image, 40,* 138–145. https://doi.org/10.1016/J.BODYIM.2021.12.006.

Demos, K. E., Kelley, W. M., & Heatherton, T. F. (2011). Dietary restraint violations influence reward responses in nucleus accumbens and amygdala. *Journal of Cognitive Neuroscience, 23*(8), 1952–1963. https://doi.org/10.1162/JOCN.2010.21568.

Denny, K. N., Loth, K., Eisenberg, M. E., & Neumark-Sztainer, D. R. (2013). Intuitive eating in young adults. Who is doing it, and how is it related to disordered eating behaviors? *Appetite, 60,* 13–19. https://doi.org/10.1016/j.appet.2012.09.029.

Diemer, E. W., White Hughto, J. M., Gordon, A. R., Guss, C., Austin, S. B., & Reisner, S. L. (2018). Beyond the binary: Differences in eating disorder prevalence by gender identity in a transgender sample. *Transgender Health, 3*(1), 17–23. https://doi.org/10.1089/trgh.2017.0043.

Dryer, R., Farr, M., Hiramatsu, I., & Quinton, S. (2016). The role of sociocultural influences on symptoms of muscle dysmorphia and eating disorders in men, and the mediating effects of perfectionism. *Behavioral Medicine, 42*(3), 174–182. https://doi.org/10.1080/08964289.2015.1122570.

Duane, A., Casimir, A. E., Mims, L. C., Kaler-Jones, C., & Simmons, D. (2021). Beyond deep breathing: A new vision for equitable, culturally responsive, and trauma-informed mindfulness practice. *Middle School Journal, 52*(3), 4–14. https://doi.org/10.1080/00940771.2021.1893593.

Dunn, T. M., & Bratman, S. (2016). On orthorexia nervosa: A review of the literature and proposed diagnostic criteria. *Eating Behaviors, 21,* 11–17. https://doi.org/10.1016/j.eatbeh.2015.12.006.

Fairburn, C. G., & Beglin, S. J. (2008). Eating Disorder Examination Questionnaire (EDE-Q 6.0). In C. G. Fairburn (Ed.), *Cognitive behavior therapy and eating disorders* (pp. 309–313). New York: Guilford Press.

Fatt, S. J., Fardouly, J., & Rapee, R. M. (2019). #malefitspo: Links between viewing fitspiration posts, muscular-ideal internalisation, appearance comparisons, body satisfaction, and exercise motivation in men. *New Media & Society, 21*(6), 1311–1325. https://doi.org/10.1177/1461444818821064.

Festinger, L. (1954). A theory of social comparison process. *Human Relations, 7*(2), 117–140. http://doi.org/10.1177/001872675400700202.

Festinger, L. (1957). *A theory of cognitive dissonance.* Redwood City, CA: Stanford University Press.

Fothergill, E., Guo, J., Howard, L., Kerns, J. C., Knuth, N. D., Brychta, R., et al. (2016). Persistent metabolic adaptation 6 years after "The Biggest Loser" competition. *Obesity, 24*(8), 1612–1619. https://doi.org/10.1002/oby.21538.

French, B. H., Lewis, J. A., Mosley, D. V., Adames, H. Y., Chavez-Dueñas, N. Y., Chen, G. A., & Neville, H. A. (2020). Toward a psychological framework of radical healing in communities of color. *The Counseling Psychologist, 48*(1), 14–46. https://doi.org/10.1177/0011000019843506.

Fuller-Tyszkiewicz, M. (2019). Body image states in everyday life: Evidence from ecological momentary assessment methodology. *Body Image, 31,* 245–272. https://doi.org/10.1016/j.bodyim.2019.02.010.

Fumagalli, M., Moltke, I., Grarup, N., Racimo, F., Bjerregaard, P., Jørgensen, M. E., et al. (2015). Greenlandic Inuit show genetic signatures of diet and climate adaptation. *Science, 349*(6254), 1343–1347. https://doi.org/10.1126/science.aab2319.

Galgani, J. E., & Santos, J. L. (2016). Insights about weight loss-induced metabolic adaptation. *Obesity, 24*(2), 277–278. https://doi.org/10.1002/oby.21408.

Galmiche, M., Déchelotte, P., Lambert, G., & Tavolacci, M. P. (2019). Prevalence of eating disorders over the 2000–2018 period: A systematic literature review. *American Journal of Clinical Nutrition, 109*(5), 1402–1413. https://doi.org/10.1093/ajcn/nqy342.

Gillespie-Smith, K., Hendry, G., Anduuru, N., Laird, T., & Ballantyne, C. (2021). Using social media to be 'social': Perceptions of social media benefits and risk by autistic young people, and parents. *Research in Developmental Disabilities, 118,* 104081. https://doi.org/10.1016/j.ridd.2021.104081.

References

Goel, N. J., Burnette, C. B., Weinstock, M., & Mazzeo, S. E. (2022). Eating Disorder Examination-Questionnaire: Evaluating factor structures and establishing measurement invariance with Asian/Hawaiian/Pacific Islander, Black, and White American college men. *International Journal of Eating Disorders, 55*(4), 481–493. https://doi.org/10.1002/EAT.23696.

Greenleaf, C., Petrie, T. A., Carter, J., & Reel, J. J. (2009). Female collegiate athletes: Prevalence of eating disorders and disordered eating behaviors. *Journal of American College Health, 57*(5), 489–496. https://doi.org/10.3200/JACH.57.5.489-496.

Grider, H. S., Douglas, S. M., & Raynor, H. A. (2021). The influence of mindful eating and/or intuitive eating approaches on dietary intake: A systematic review. *Journal of the Academy of Nutrition and Dietetics, 121*(4), 709–727. https://doi.org/10.1016/j.jand.2020.10.019.

Grilo, C. M., Ivezaj, V., & White, M. A. (2015). Evaluation of the DSM-5 severity indicator for binge eating disorder in a clinical sample. *Behaviour Research and Therapy, 71*, 110–114. https://doi.org/10.1016/j.brat.2015.05.003.

Hahn, S. L., Barry, M. R., Weeks, H. M., Miller, A. L., Lumeng, J. C., & Sonneville, K. R. (2021). Parental perceptions of actual and ideal body weight in early childhood prospectively predict adolescent perceptions of actual and ideal body weight among a low-income population. *Eating and Weight Disorders, 26*(7), 2371–2379. https://doi.org/10.1007%2Fs40519-020-01088-y.

Hahn, S. L., Burnette, C. B., Hooper, L., Wall, M., Loth, K. A., & Neumark-Sztainer, D. (2023). Do weight perception transitions in adolescence predict concurrent and long-term disordered eating behaviors? *Journal of Adolescent Health, 72*(5), 803–810. https://doi.org/10.1016/j.jadohealth.2022.12.023.

Hall, K. D., & Guo, J. (2017). Obesity energetics: Body weight regulation and the effects of diet composition. *Gastroenterology, 152*(7), 1718-1727.e3. https://doi.org/10.1053/j.gastro.2017.01.052.

Hansen, A. W., Christensen, D. L., Larsson, M. W., Eis, J., Christensen, T., Friis, H., et al. (2011). Dietary patterns, food and macronutrient intakes among adults in three ethnic groups in rural Kenya. *Public Health Nutrition, 14*(9), 1671–1679. https://doi.org/10.1017/S1368980010003782.

Harriger, J. A., Evans, J. A., Thompson, J. K., & Tylka, T. L. (2022). The dangers of the rabbit hole: Reflections on social media as a portal into a distorted world of edited bodies and eating disorder risk and the role of algorithms. *Body Image, 41*, 292–297. https://doi.org/10.1016/j.bodyim.2022.03.007.

Harriger, J. A., Thompson, J. K., & Tiggemann, M. (2023). TikTok, TikTok, the time is now: Future directions in social media and body image. *Body Image, 44*, 222–226. https://doi.org/10.1016/j.bodyim.2023.01.005.

Harrison, D. L. (2021). *Belly of the beast: The politics of anti-fatness as anti-Blackness*. Berkeley, CA: North Atlantic Books.

Hart, L. M., Granillo, M. T., Jorm, A. F., & Paxton, S. J. (2011). Unmet need for treatment in the eating disorders: A systematic review of eating disorder specific treatment seeking among community cases. *Clinical Psychology Review, 31*(5), 727–735. https://doi.org/10.1016/j.cpr.2011.03.004.

Hartman-Munick, S. M., Silverstein, S., Guss, C. E., Lopez, E., Calzo, J. P., & Gordon, A. R. (2021). Eating disorder screening and treatment experiences in transgender and gender diverse young adults. *Eating Behaviors, 41*, 101517. https://doi.org/10.1016/j.eatbeh.2021.101517.

Hatfield, T. R., Brown, R. F., Giummarra, M. J., & Lenggenhager, B. (2019). Autism spectrum disorder and interoception: Abnormalities in global integration? *Autism, 23*(1), 212–222. https://doi.org/10.1177/1362361317738392.

Hawkins, M., & Panzera, A. (2021). Food insecurity: A key determinant of health. *Archives of Psychiatric Nursing, 35*(1), 113–117. https://doi.org/10.1016/j.apnu.2020.10.011.

Hawks, S., Madanat, H., Hawks, J., & Harris, A. (2005). The relationship between intuitive eating and health indicators among college women. *American Journal of Health Education, 36*(6), 331–336. https://doi.org/10.1080/19325037.2005.10608206.

Hawley, G., Horwath, C., Gray, A., Bradshaw, A., Katzer, L., Joyce, J., & O'Brien, S. (2008). Sustainability of health and lifestyle improvements following a non-dieting randomised trial in overweight women. *Preventive Medicine, 47*(6), 593–599. https://doi.org/10.1016/j.ypmed.2008.08.008.

Hazzard, V. M., Burnette, C. B., Hooper, L., Larson, N., Eisenberg, M. E., & Neumark-Sztainer, D. (2022). Lifestyle health behavior correlates of intuitive eating in a population-based sample of men and women. *Eating Behaviors, 46*, 101644. https://doi.org/10.1016/j.eatbeh.2022.101644.

Hazzard, V. M., Loth, K. A., Hooper, L., & Becker, C. B. (2020). Food insecurity and eating disorders: A review of emerging evidence. *Current Psychiatry Reports, 22*(12), 1–9. https://doi.org/10.1007/S11920-020-01200-0.

Hazzard, V. M., Telke, S. E., Simone, M., Anderson, L. M., Larson, N. I., & Neumark-Sztainer, D. R. (2021). Intuitive eating longitudinally predicts better psychological health and lower use of disordered eating behaviors: Findings from EAT 2010–2018. *Eating and Weight Disorders—Studies on Anorexia, Bulimia and Obesity, 26*, 287–294. https://doi.org/10.1007/s40519-020-00852-4.

Hensley-Hackett, K., Bosker, J., Keefe, A., Reidlinger, D., Warner, M., D'Arcy, A., & Utter, J. (2022). Intuitive eating intervention and diet quality in adults: A systematic literature review. *Journal of Nutrition Education and Behavior, 54*(12), 1099–1115. https://doi.org/10.1016/j.jneb.2022.08.008.

Holtzman, B., & Ackerman, K. E. (2019). Measurement, determinants, and implications of energy intake in athletes. *Nutrients, 11*(3), Article 3. https://doi.org/10.3390/nu11030665.

Hunter, E. A., Kluck, A. S., Ramon, A. E., Ruff, E., & Dario, J. (2020). The Curvy Ideal Silhouette Scale: Measuring cultural differences in the body shape ideals of young U.S. women. *Sex Roles, 84*, 238–251. https://doi.org/10.1007/s11199-020-01161-x.

Huryk, K. M., Drury, C. R., & Loeb, K. L. (2021). Diseases of affluence? A systematic review of the literature on socioeconomic diversity in eating disorders. *Eating Behaviors, 43*, 101548. https://doi.org/10.1016/j.eatbeh.2021.101548.

Iijima Hall, C. C. (1995). Asian eyes: Body image and eating disorders of Asian and Asian American women. *Eating Disorders, 3*(1), 8–19. https://doi.org/10.1080/10640269508249141.

Jackson, A., Sano, Y., Parker, L., Cox, A. E., & Lanigan, J. (2022). Intuitive eating and dietary intake. *Eating Behaviors, 45*, 101606. https://doi.org/10.1016/J.EATBEH.2022.101606.

Kamody, R. C., Grilo, C. M., & Udo, T. (2020). Disparities in DSM-5 defined eating disorders by sexual orientation among U.S. adults. *International Journal of Eating Disorders, 53*(2), 278–287. https://doi.org/10.1002/eat.23193.

Kawano, H., Mineta, M., Asaka, M., Miyashita, M., Numao, S., Gando, Y., Ando, T., Sakamoto, S., & Higuchi, M. (2013). Effects of different modes of exercise on appetite and appetite-regulating hormones. *Appetite, 66*, 26–33. https://doi.org/10.1016/j.appet.2013.01.017.

Kelly, A. (2015). Trauma-informed mindfulness-based stress reduction: A promising new model for working with survivors of interpersonal violence. *Smith College Studies in Social Work, 85*(2), 194–219. https://doi.org/10.1080/00377317.2015.1021191.

Kini, P., Wong, J., McInnis, S., Gabana, N., & Brown, J. W. (2016). The effects of gratitude expression on neural activity. *NeuroImage, 128*, 1–10. https://doi.org/10.1016/j.neuroimage.2015.12.040.

Kivlighan, D. M., Jr., London, K., & Miles, J. R. (2012). Are two heads better than one? The relationship between number of group leaders and group members, and group climate and group member benefit from therapy. *Group Dynamics: Theory, Research, and Practice, 16*, 1–13. https://doi.org/10.1037/a0026242.

Kutscheidt, K., Dresler, T., Hudak, J., Barth, B., Blume, F., Ethofer, T., et al. (2019). Interoceptive awareness in patients with attention-deficit/hyperactivity disorder (ADHD). *ADHD Attention Deficit and Hyperactivity Disorders, 11*(4), 395–401. https://doi.org/10.1007/s12402-019-00299-3.

Lavender, J. M., Brown, T. A., & Murray, S. B. (2017). Men, muscles, and eating disorders: An overview of traditional and muscularity-oriented disordered eating. *Current Psychiatry Reports, 19*(6), 1–7. https://doi.org/10.1007/s11920-017-0787-5.

References

Linardon, J., Messer, M., Helms, E. R., McLean, C., Incerti, L., & Fuller-Tyszkiewicz, M. (2020). Interactions between different eating patterns on recurrent binge-eating behavior: A machine learning approach. *International Journal of Eating Disorders*, 53(4), 533–540. https://doi.org/10.1002/EAT.23232.

Linardon, J., Tylka, T. L., & Fuller-Tyszkiewicz, M. (2021). Intuitive eating and its psychological correlates: A meta-analysis. *International Journal of Eating Disorders*, 54(7), 1073–1098. https://doi.org/10.1002/EAT.23509.

Lipson, S. K., & Sonneville, K. R. (2017). Eating disorder symptoms among undergraduate and graduate students at 12 U.S. colleges and universities. *Eating Behaviors*, 24, 81–88. https://doi.org/10.1016/j.eatbeh.2016.12.003.

Lopez, T. D., Hernandez, D., Bode, S., & Ledoux, T. (2023). A complex relationship between intuitive eating and diet quality among university students. *Journal of American College Health*, 71(9), 2751–2757. https://doi.org/10.1080/07448481.2021.1996368.

Loth, K. A., MacLehose, R., Bucchianeri, M., Crow, S., & Neumark-Sztainer, D. R. (2014). Predictors of dieting and disordered eating behaviors from adolescence to young adulthood. *Journal of Adolescent Health*, 55(5), 705–712. https://doi.org/10.1016/j.jadohealth.2014.04.016.

MacLean, P. S., Higgins, J. A., Johnson, G. C., Fleming-Elder, B. K., Donahoo, W. T., Melanson, E. L., & Hill, J. O. (2004). Enhanced metabolic efficiency contributes to weight regain after weight loss in obesity-prone rats. *American Journal of Physiology-Regulatory, Integrative and Comparative Physiology*, 287(6), R1306–R1315. https://doi.org/10.1152/ajpregu.00463.2004.

Madden, C. E., Leong, S. L., Gray, A., & Horwath, C. C. (2012). Eating in response to hunger and satiety signals is related to BMI in a nationwide sample of 1601 mid-age New Zealand women. *Public Health Nutrition*, 15(12), 2272–2279. https://doi.org/10.1017/S1368980012000882.

Mancine, R. P., Gusfa, D. W., Moshrefi, A., & Kennedy, S. F. (2020). Prevalence of disordered eating in athletes categorized by emphasis on leanness and activity type—A systematic review. *Journal of Eating Disorders*, 8(1), 47. https://doi.org/10.1186/s40337-020-00323-2.

Mann, T., Tomiyama, A. J., Westling, E., Lew, A.-M., Samuels, B., & Chatman, J. (2007). Medicare's search for effective obesity treatments: Diets are not the answer. *American Psychologist*, 62(3), 220–233. https://doi.org/10.1037/0003-066X.62.3.220.

Marks, R. J., De Foe, A., & Collett, J. (2020). The pursuit of wellness: Social media, body image and eating disorders. *Children and Youth Services Review*, 119, 105659. https://doi.org/10.1016/j.childyouth.2020.105659.

Meadows, A., & Daníelsdóttir, S. (2016). What's in a word? On weight stigma and terminology. *Frontiers in Psychology*, 7, 1–4. https://doi.org/10.3389/fpsyg.2016.01527.

Meneguzzo, P., Collantoni, E., Gallicchio, D., Busetto, P., Solmi, M., Santonastaso, P., & Favaro, A. (2018). Eating disorders symptoms in sexual minority women: A systematic review. *European Eating Disorders Review*, 26(4), 275–292. https://doi.org/10.1002/erv.2601.

Mensinger, J. L., Calogero, R. M., Stranges, S., & Tylka, T. L. (2016). A weight-neutral versus weight-loss approach for health promotion in women with high BMI: A randomized-controlled trial. *Appetite*, 105, 364–374. https://doi.org/10.1016/j.appet.2016.06.006.

Moltke, I., Grarup, N., Jørgensen, M. E., Bjerregaard, P., Treebak, J. T., Fumagalli, M., et al. (2014). A common Greenlandic TBC1D4 variant confers muscle insulin resistance and type 2 diabetes. *Nature*, 512(7513), Article 7513. https://doi.org/10.1038/nature13425.

Mond, J. M., Latner, J. D., Hay, P. H., Owen, C., & Rodgers, B. (2010). Objective and subjective bulimic episodes in the classification of bulimic-type eating disorders: Another nail in the coffin of a problematic distinction. *Behaviour Research and Therapy*, 48(7), 661–669. https://doi.org/10.1016/j.brat.2010.03.020.

Mountjoy, M., Sundgot-Borgen, J., Burke, L., Carter, S., Constantini, N., Lebrun, C., et al. (2014). The IOC consensus statement: Beyond the Female Athlete Triad—Relative Energy Deficiency in Sport (RED-S). *British Journal of Sports Medicine*, 48(7), 491–497. https://doi.org/10.1136/bjsports-2014-093502.

Naslund, J. A., Bondre, A., Torous, J., & Aschbrenner, K. A. (2020). Social media and mental health: Benefits, risks, and opportunities for research and practice. *Journal of Technology in Behavioral Science, 5*(3), 245–257. https://doi.org/10.1007/s41347-020-00134-x.

Nechita, D.-M., Bud, S., & David, D. (2021). Shame and eating disorders symptoms: A meta-analysis. *International Journal of Eating Disorders, 54*(11), 1899–1945. https://doi.org/10.1002/eat.23583.

Nordmo, M., Danielsen, Y. S., & Nordmo, M. (2020). The challenge of keeping it off, a descriptive systematic review of high-quality, follow-up studies of obesity treatments. *Obesity Reviews, 21*(1), e12949. https://doi.org/10.1111/obr.12949.

Owen, P. R., & Laurel-Seller, E. (2000). Weight and shape ideals: Thin is dangerously in. *Journal of Applied Social Psychology, 30*(5), 979–990. https://doi.org/10.1111/j.1559-1816.2000.tb02506.x.

Panza, E., Fehling, K. B., Pantalone, D. W., Dodson, S., & Selby, E. A. (2021). Multiply marginalized: Linking minority stress due to sexual orientation, gender, and weight to dysregulated eating among sexual minority women of higher body weight. *Psychology of Sexual Orientation and Gender Diversity, 8*(4), 420–428. https://doi.org/10.1037/SGD0000431.

Petrie, T. A., & Greenleaf, C. A. (2007). Eating disorders in sport: From theory to research to intervention. In G. Tenenbaum & R. C. Eklund (Eds.), *Handbook of sport psychology* (3rd ed., pp. 352–378). Hoboken, NJ: John Wiley & Sons.

Pew Research Center. (2021). Social media fact sheet. *Pew Research Center: Internet, Science & Tech*. Retrieved April 22, 2023, from https://www.pewresearch.org/internet/fact-sheet/social-media.

Piran, N. (2016). Embodied possibilities and disruptions: The emergence of the Experience of Embodiment construct from qualitative studies with girls and women. *Body Image, 18*, 43–60. https://doi.org/10.1016/j.bodyim.2016.04.007.

Prichard, I., Kavanagh, E., Mulgrew, K. E., Lim, M. S. C., & Tiggemann, M. (2020). The effect of Instagram #fitspiration images on young women's mood, body image, and exercise behaviour. *Body Image, 33*, 1–6. https://doi.org/10.1016/j.bodyim.2020.02.002.

Puhl, R. M., Latner, J. D., O'Brien, K. S., Luedicke, J., Danielsdottir, S., & Forhan, M. (2015). A multinational examination of weight bias: Predictors of anti-fat attitudes across four countries. *International Journal of Obesity, 39*, 1166–1173.

Quansah, D. Y., Gilbert, L., Gross, J., Horsch, A., & Puder, J. J. (2019). Intuitive eating is associated with improved health indicators at 1-year postpartum in women with gestational diabetes mellitus. *Journal of Health Psychology, 26*(8), 1168–1184. https://doi.org/10.1177/1359105319869814.

Räisänen, U., & Hunt, K. (2014). The role of gendered constructions of eating disorders in delayed help-seeking in men: A qualitative interview study. *BMJ Open, 4*(4), e004342. https://doi.org/10.1136/bmjopen-2013-004342.

Resch, E. (2019). *The intuitive eating workbook for teens: A non-diet, body positive approach to building a healthy relationship with food*. Oakland, CA: Instant Help.

Rodgers, R. F., Paxton, S. J., & Wertheim, E. H. (2021). #Take idealized bodies out of the picture: A scoping review of social media content aiming to protect and promote positive body image. *Body Image, 38*, 10–36. https://doi.org/10.1016/j.bodyim.2021.03.009.

Rodin, J., Silberstein, L. R., & Striegel-Moore, R. (1985). Women and weight: A normative discontent. In T. Sondergger (Ed.), *Psychology and gender: Nebraska symposium on motivation* (pp. 206–237). Lincoln, NE: University of Nebraska Press.

Root, M. P. P. (1990). Disordered eating in women of color. *Sex Roles, 22*(7–8), 525–536. https://doi.org/10.1007/BF00288168.

Rubino, F., Puhl, R. M., Cummings, D. E., Eckel, R. H., Ryan, D. H., Mechanick, J. I., et al. (2020). Joint international consensus statement for ending stigma of obesity. *Nature Medicine, 26*(4), 485–497. https://doi.org/10.1038/s41591-020-0803-x.

Samuels, K. L., Maine, M. M., & Tantillo, M. (2019). Disordered eating, eating disorders, and body image in midlife and older women. *Current Psychiatry Reports, 21*(8), 70. https://doi.org/10.1007/s11920-019-1057-5.

References

Satterfield, N. A., & Stutts, L. A. (2021). Pinning down the problems and influences: Disordered eating and body satisfaction in male wrestlers. *Psychology of Sport and Exercise, 54*, 101884. https://doi.org/10.1016/j.psychsport.2021.101884.

Schooler, D., & Daniels, E. A. (2014). "I am not a skinny toothpick and proud of it": Latina adolescents' ethnic identity and responses to mainstream media images. *Body Image, 11*(1), 11–18. https://doi.org/10.1016/J.BODYIM.2013.09.001.

Serier, K. N., Smith, J. E., & Yeater, E. A. (2018). Confirmatory factor analysis and measurement invariance of the Eating Disorder Examination Questionnaire (EDE-Q) in a non-clinical sample of non-Hispanic White and Hispanic women. *Eating Behaviors, 31*, 53–59. https://doi.org/10.1016/j.eatbeh.2018.08.004.

Shigekawa, E., Fix, M., Corbett, G., Roby, D. H., & Coffman, J. (2018). The current state of telehealth evidence: A rapid review. *Health Affairs, 37*(12), 1975–1982. https://doi.org/10.1377/hlthaff.2018.05132.

Smolak, L., & Striegel-Moore, R. H. (2004). Challenging the myth of the golden girl: Ethnicity and eating disorders. In R. H. Striegel-Moore & L. Smolak (Eds.), *Eating disorders: Innovative directions in research and practice* (pp. 111–132). Washington, DC: American Psychological Association. https://doi.org/10.1037/10403-006.

Snoswell, C. L., Chelberg, G., De Guzman, K. R., Haydon, H. H., Thomas, E. E., Caffery, L. J., & Smith, A. C. (2021). The clinical effectiveness of telehealth: A systematic review of meta-analyses from 2010 to 2019. *Journal of Telemedicine and Telecare, 29*(9), 669–684. https://doi.org/10.1177/1357633X211022907.

Sonneville, K. R., & Lipson, S. K. (2018). Disparities in eating disorder diagnosis and treatment according to weight status, race/ethnicity, socioeconomic background, and sex among college students. *International Journal of Eating Disorders, 51*, 518–526. https://doi.org/10.1002/eat.22846.

Spirou, D., Raman, J., & Smith, E. (2020). Psychological outcomes following surgical and endoscopic bariatric procedures: A systematic review. *Obesity Reviews, 21*(6), e12998. https://doi.org/10.1111/obr.12998.

Steiger, H., Booij, L., Crescenzi, O., Oliverio, S., Singer, I., Thaler, L., et al. (2022). In-person versus virtual therapy in outpatient eating-disorder treatment: A COVID-19 inspired study. *International Journal of Eating Disorders, 55*(1), 145–150. https://doi.org/10.1002/eat.23655.

Steinberg, D. M., Perry, T. R., Freestone, D., Hellner, M., Baker, J. H., & Bohon, C. (2023). Evaluating differences in setting expected body weight for children and adolescents in eating disorder treatment. *International Journal of Eating Disorders, 56*(3), 595–603. https://doi.org/10.1002/eat.23868.

Stice, E., Burger, K., & Yokum, S. (2013). Caloric deprivation increases responsivity of attention and reward brain regions to intake, anticipated intake, and images of palatable foods. *NeuroImage, 67*, 322–330. https://doi.org/10.1016/j.neuroimage.2012.11.028.

Striegel-Moore, R. H., Silberstein, L. R., Frensch, P., & Rodin, J. (1989). A prospective study of disordered eating among college students. *International Journal of Eating Disorders, 8*(5), 499–509. https://doi.org/10.1002/1098-108X(198909)8:5%3C499::AID-EAT2260080502%3E3.0.CO;2-A.

Strings, S. (2019). *Fearing the Black body: The racial origins of fat phobia*. New York: New York University Press.

Strother, E., Lemberg, R., Stanford, S. C., & Turberville, D. (2012). Eating disorders in men: Underdiagnosed, undertreated, and misunderstood. *Eating Disorders, 20*(5), 346–355. https://doi.org/10.1080/10640266.2012.715512.

Tay, L., & Diener, E. (2011). Needs and subjective well-being around the world. *Journal of Personality and Social Psychology, 101*, 354–365. https://doi.org/10.1037/a0023779.

Thomas, J. J., Becker, K. R., & Eddy, K. T. (2021). *The picky eater's recovery book: Overcoming avoidant/restrictive food intake disorder*. New York: Cambridge University Press.

Thomas, J. J., & Eddy, K. T. (2018). *Cognitive-behavioral therapy for avoidant/restrictive food intake disorder: Children, adolescents, and adults.* New York: Cambridge University Press.

Tomiyama, A. J. (2014). Weight stigma is stressful. A review of evidence for the Cyclic Obesity/Weight-Based Stigma model. *Appetite, 82,* 8–15. https://doi.org/10.1016/j.appet.2014.06.108.

Tomiyama, A. J., Mann, T., Vinas, D., Hunger, J. M., DeJager, J., & Taylor, S. E. (2010). Low calorie dieting increases cortisol. *Psychosomatic Medicine, 72*(4), 357–364. https://doi.org/10.1097/PSY.0b013e3181d9523c.

Tordoff, D. M., Wanta, J. W., Collin, A., Stepney, C., Inwards-Breland, D. J., & Ahrens, K. (2022). Mental health outcomes in transgender and nonbinary youths receiving gender-affirming care. *JAMA Network Open, 5*(2), e220978. https://doi.org/10.1001/jamanetworkopen.2022.0978.

Torous, J., Bucci, S., Bell, I. H., Kessing, L. V., Faurholt-Jepsen, M., Whelan, P., et al. (2021). The growing field of digital psychiatry: Current evidence and the future of apps, social media, chatbots, and virtual reality. *World Psychiatry, 20*(3), 318–335. https://doi.org/10.1002/WPS.20883.

Traviss-Turner, G. D., West, R. M., & Hill, A. J. (2017). Guided self-help for eating disorders: A systematic review and metaregression. *European Eating Disorders Review, 25*(3), 148–164. https://doi.org/10.1002/erv.2507.

Tribole, E., & Resch, E. (2017). *The intuitive eating workbook: Ten principles for nourishing a healthy relationship with food.* Oakland, CA: New Harbinger Publications.

Tribole, E., & Resch, E. (2020). *Intuitive eating: A revolutionary program that works.* New York: St. Martin's Griffin.

Turner, P. G., & Lefevre, C. E. (2017). Instagram use is linked to increased symptoms of orthorexia nervosa. *Eating and Weight Disorders—Studies on Anorexia, Bulimia and Obesity, 22*(2), 277–284. https://doi.org/10.1007/s40519-017-0364-2.

Tylka, T., Fuller-Tyszkiewicz, M., Swami, V., Burnette, C. B., Todd, J., & Linardon, J. (2023). *Intuitive Eating Scale-3: Development and psychometric investigation.* https://doi.org/10.17605/OSF.IO/8T7ZM.

Tylka, T. L., Calogero, R. M., & Mensinger, J. L. (2019). Pressure to be thin and body acceptance by others mediate the relationship between BMI and intuitive eating. *International Conference on Eating Disorders.*

Tylka, T. L., & Homan, K. J. (2015). Exercise motives and positive body image in physically active college women and men: Exploring an expanded acceptance model of intuitive eating. *Body Image, 15,* 90–97. https://doi.org/10.1016/j.bodyim.2015.07.003.

Tylka, T. L., & Kroon Van Diest, A. M. (2013). The Intuitive Eating Scale–2: Item refinement and psychometric evaluation with college women and men. *Journal of Counseling Psychology, 60*(1), 137–153. https://doi.org/10.1037/a0030893.

Tylka, T. L., & Kroon Van Diest, A. M. (2015). Protective factors. In L. Smolak & M. P. Levine (Eds.), *The Wiley Handbook of Eating Disorders* (pp. 430–444). Chichester, UK: Wiley Blackwell. https://doi.org/10.1002/9781118574089.ch33.

Tylka, T. L., & Wood-Barcalow, N. L. (2015). What is and what is not positive body image? Conceptual foundations and construct definition. *Body Image, 14,* 118–129. https://doi.org/10.1016/j.bodyim.2015.04.001.

Van Dam, N. T., van Vugt, M. K., Vago, D. R., Schmalzl, L., Saron, C. D., Olendzki, A., et al. (2018). Mind the hype: A critical evaluation and prescriptive agenda for research on mindfulness and meditation. *Perspectives on Psychological Science, 13*(1), 36–61. https://doi.org/10.1177/1745691617709589.

Van Dyke, N., & Drinkwater, E. J. (2014). Relationships between intuitive eating and health indicators: Literature review. *Public Health Nutrition, 17*(8), 1757–1766. https://doi.org/10.1017/S1368980013002139.

Vartanian, L. R., Wharton, C. M., & Green, E. B. (2012). Appearance vs. health motives for exercise and for weight loss. *Psychology of Sport and Exercise, 13*(3), 251–256. https://doi.org/10.1016/j.psychsport.2011.12.005.

Blair Burnette, PhD, is assistant professor in the psychology department at Michigan State University. She has published nearly forty peer-reviewed articles on social and cultural factors that contribute to body image concerns, disordered eating, and eating disorders—with a particular focus on intuitive eating. Burnette serves on the editorial board of the journal *Body Image*, and is an active committee member of the Academy for Eating Disorders. She is from Nashville, TN.

Foreword writer **Tracy L. Tylka, PhD**, is professor of psychology at The Ohio State University. Tylka is a fellow of the Academy for Eating Disorders, and editor of *Body Image*.

Index

NUMBERS
27-item intuitive eating scale, 13

A
ableist language, 140
acceptance and commitment therapy, 15, 91–93
acceptance model, 12, 31
alexithymia, 9, 123
algorithms, social media, 135
Alleva, Jessica, 131
ANAD Recovery Mentorship Program, 175
anorexia nervosa, 23
anti-fat bias, 21–22
appreciation, 131
ARFID (avoidant/restrictive food intake disorder), 25, 106
assessments, 37–38
assumptions, 19–20
athletes
    benefits of and barriers to intuitive movement, 145–146
    considerations for working with, 27–28
    relationship with movement, 140
autism. *see* neurodivergent populations
avoidant/restrictive food intake disorder (ARFID), 25, 106

B
beauty ideals, 21
BED (binge eating disorder), 23–24
Bennett, Brooke, 24
between-session exercises
    celebrating progress session, 168
    Challenge the Food Police principle, 89–90, 96–97
    Cope with Your Emotions with Kindness principle, 115–116, 122
    debriefing, 38–39
    Discover the Satisfaction Factor principle, 101–102, 111
    Feel Your Fullness principle, 101–102, 111
    Honor Your Health—Gentle Nutrition principle, 163–164
    Honor Your Hunger principle, 65, 70
    Make Peace with Food principle, 75–76, 85
    Movement—Feel the Difference principle, 141, 148
    Reject Diet Culture principle, 59–60
    Respect Your Body principle, 126–127, 136
    review of assigned, 39–40
biases, 20, 125, 135
Biggest Loser contestants, 53
binge eating, 22–23, 65
binge eating disorder (BED), 23–24
biological hunger, 66–67
BMI (body mass index), 18, 50
body image concerns, 20–22. *see also* Respect Your Body principle
    cultivating body respect, 130–133
    ditching dieting and, 47
    life without body negativity, 129–130
    responding to body talk, 133–135
body image–related distress, 21
body mass index (BMI), 18, 50
body positivity, 31
Body Project, 32
body–food choice congruence, 154–155
body-neutral communities, 31
Borton, Kelley, 25–26
bounds, eating, 77–80
bulimia nervosa, 23
bulking behavior, 51

C
carbohydrates, 108, 152
Challenge the Food Police principle, 8–9, 87–98
    closing sessions, 97
    considerations and adaptations, 89
    expectations of session, 88–89
    overview, 90–94

responding to food-related comments, 94–96
session aim, 88
between-session exercises, 89–90, 96–97
chronic dieting, 22
chronic illnesses, 140
chronic stress, 69
Cichy, Meghan, 27
Clark, Christine, 28
clients, 19–29
   body image concerns, 20–22
   chronic or yo-yo dieting, 22
   dietary restrictions and modifications, 26–27
   disordered eating and eating disorders, 22–24
   incorporating gentle nutrition, 157–158
   needing more time, 175–176
   not ready to incorporate intuitive eating, 25–26
   ready to incorporate intuitive eating, 24–25
   stigma, stereotypes, and assumptions, 19–20
   trauma, 29
   working with athletes, 27–28
closed groups, 34
closing sessions, 40
   Challenge the Food Police principle, 97
   Cope with Your Emotions with Kindness principle, 122
   Discover the Satisfaction Factor principle, 111
   Feel Your Fullness principle, 111
   Honor Your Health—Gentle Nutrition principle, 164
   Honor Your Hunger principle, 70
   Make Peace with Food principle, 85
   Movement—Feel the Difference principle, 148
   Reject Diet Culture principle, 60
   Respect Your Body principle, 136
cognitive behavioral therapy, 91–93
cognitive dissonance theory, 32
cognitive manifestations of hunger, 67
cognitive restructuring, 9
co-led groups, 34

comparisons, social, 75, 89
compensatory exercise, 22–23, 143, 147–148
compulsive exercise, 22–23, 147–148
contentment, 110
co-occurring diagnoses, 176
Cope with Your Emotions with Kindness principle, 9, 113–123
   checking in on self-care, 117–118
   closing sessions, 122
   considerations and adaptations, 114–115
   cultivating new coping strategies, 120–122
   exercise behaviors, 118–119
   role of emotions in eating, 116–117
   session aim, 114
   between-session exercises, 115–116, 122
cravings, 110
curiosity, encouraging, 49, 160–162

D

David, Susan, 120
dialectical behavior therapy, 120
diet pill use, 22–23
dietary quality, 15–17
dietary restraint theory, 8
dietitians, 26
diets. *see also* Reject Diet Culture principle
   defined, 46, 52–53
   identifying problem with, 53–54
   rejecting diet culture, 8, 171
   reluctance to let go of, 57–58
   restrictions and modifications, 26–27
disabilities, 140
Discover the Satisfaction Factor principle, 9, 99–112
   barriers to feeling and honoring fullness, 104–108
   closing sessions, 111
   considerations and adaptations, 100–101
   discovering staying power of foods, 108–109
   feeling fullness overview, 102–104
   overview, 109–111
   session aim, 100
   between-session exercises, 101–102, 111
disease risk, 73
disordered eating, 13–15, 22–24
   athletes with, 27–28

Index

habituation fears, 84
neurodivergent populations with, 74
social media causing risk of, 135
disordered muscle-building behaviors, 22–23
dissonance-based exercises, 54, 82–83
distracted eating, 105–106
diuretic misuse, 22–23
diversity, body, 127–128
doctor visits, 132
downward comparisons, 32

E

early satiety, 105
eating
behaviors, 14–15
emotional eating, 114
micromanaging, 56–59
Eating Disorder Examination, 38
eating disorders, 22–24
ditching dieting session considerations, 47
habituation fears, 84
micromanaging eating, 56
open weighing, 50
Emotional Agility (David), 120
emotional eating, 9
defined, 114
functions and consequences of, 118–119
identifying, 117–118
emotion-focused coping, 121
emotions. *see* Cope with Your Emotions with Kindness principle
empathy, 55
endurance athletes, 27
enhanced cognitive behavioral therapy, 58, 176
evidence base, 11–18
measurement of intuitive eating, 13
models of intuitive eating, 12–13
research, 13–18
exercise, 17. *see also* Movement—Feel the Difference principle
movement versus, 141–142
role of emotions in, 118–119
exposure exercises, 83
exposure mindset, 24

F

fat clients, 21

fats, 108
fear
of fullness, 106
habituation fears, 84–85
fear-avoidance cycle, 81–82
FEDUP Collective, 175
Feel Your Fullness principle, 9, 99–112
barriers to feeling and honoring fullness, 104–108
closing sessions, 111
considerations and adaptations, 100–101
discovering staying power of foods, 108–109
overview, 102–104
satisfaction factor overview, 109–111
session aim, 100
between-session exercises, 101–102, 111
fight-or-flight response, 69
filtering content, 135
fitspiration, 139
flexible dietary control, 14–15
food. *see also* Honor Your Health—Gentle Nutrition principle; Make Peace with Food principle
choosing less satisfying, 105
discovering staying power of, 108–109
forbidden foods, 16–17
rules, 76–80
What Is Food For? exercise, 162–163
food-related beliefs
evaluating, 91–93
exploring, 90–91
responding to comments about, 94–96
fullness. *see also* Feel Your Fullness principle
barriers to feeling and honoring, 104–108
cultivating awareness of, 26–27
exploring patterns with clients, 115–116
Feel Your Fullness principle, 9
overview, 102–104

G

gender dysphoria, 21, 73, 114, 126
gentle nutrition. *see* Honor Your Health—Gentle Nutrition principle
glycogen stores, 27
graduated exposure, 83, 106
gratitude, 130–131

group sessions, 33–35
    body image concerns, 126
    celebrating progress session, 168
    challenging thought patterns, 89
    ditching dieting session considerations, 48
    emotional eating, 115
    finding joy in movement, 140
    finding peace with food session, 75, 79–80
    gentle nutrition, 153
    paired snack activity, 101
    sharing reasons for joining in, 64
Growing as an Intuitive Eater Plan, 167–174
growth mindset, 159–163
guided self-help, 35–36

H

habituation, 81–85
Health at Every Size, 11, 15
health behaviors and nutrition, 14–17
    dietary quality, 15–17
    eating behaviors, 14–15
    physical activity, 17
Health-focused, Understanding lifestyle, Group-supported, and Self-esteem building (HUGS), 15
Healthy Eating Index, 16
heterogeneity of group, 34–35
higher weight bodies, 21
homogeneity of group, 34–35
Honor Your Health—Gentle Nutrition principle, 10, 150–165
    closing sessions, 164
    considerations and adaptations, 152
    determing if clients are ready to incorporate, 157–158
    language shaping attitude toward food, 156–157
    overview, 154–155
    pursuit of progress over perfection, 159–163
    session aim, 151
    between-session exercises, 153–154, 163–164
Honor Your Hunger principle, 8, 62–71
    body-cue awareness, 66–67
    closing sessions, 70
    considerations and adaptations, 63–64
    distinguishing hunger cues from thoughts, 68–69
    expectations of session, 63
    hunger defined, 65–66
    self-care, 69–70
    session aim, 63
    between-session exercises, 65, 70
    signs of hunger, 67–68
HUGS (Health-focused, Understanding lifestyle, Group-supported, and Self-esteem building), 15
hunger
    athletes and cues for, 27
    body-cue awareness of, 66–67
    defined, 65–66
    distinguishing thoughts from, 68–69
    honoring, 8
    signs of, 67–68
Hunger Discovery Log, 68, 75
Hunger Rating Scale, 68, 103

I

IES-2 (Intuitive Eating Scale-2), 13, 37
individual sessions, 33, 78–79
intake process, 37
interoceptive awareness, 8
    diminished or altered, 63–64
    fullness cues, 106–107
    ultra-processed foods and, 156
intersectional identities, 20
intuitive eating, 7–18
    clients not ready to incorporate, 25–26
    clients ready to incorporate, 24–25
    conceptualization of, 10–11
    evidence base for, 11–18
    framework overview, 48–49
    principles of, 8–10
intuitive eating interventions, 30–44
    considerations for changing the session order, 44
    getting started, 36–38
    intervention modality, 33–36
    intervention structure, 30–31
    lengthening treatment, 42–44
    session structure, 38–41
    shortening treatment, 41–42
    theoretical framework, 31–32

Index

when clients need more time, 175–176
Intuitive Eating Scale-2 (IES-2), 13, 37
Intuitive Eating (Tribole and Resch), 11
The Intuitive Eating Workbook (Tribole & Resch), 35
intuitive movement, 142–144

J
junk foods, 156

K
kindness. *see* Cope with Your Emotions with Kindness principle

L
language, shaping attitude toward food, 156–157
lateral comparisons, 32
laxative abuse, 22–23
lengthening treatment, 42–44
LGBTQ, 19. *see also* gender dysphoria
lifestyle programs, 46

M
macronutrients, 108, 110
mainstream media, 10
Make Peace with Food principle, 8, 72–86
    closing sessions, 85
    considerations and adaptations, 73–74
    expectations of session, 74
    habituation, 81–85
    overview, 76–80
    session aim, 73
    between-session exercises, 75–76, 85
marginalized groups, 19, 89, 114
meal timing, 107–108
measurement of intuitive eating, 13
medically necessary dietary restrictions, 26–27, 152
men
    body image pressures with, 21, 125–126
    eating concerns with, 20
mental health, 107
metabolic adaptations, 128
micromanaging eating, 56–59
mindful eating, 11
modality, intervention, 33–36
    group sessions, 33–35
    guided self-help, 35–36
    individual sessions, 33
    involving significant others, 36
    telehealth, 36
models of intuitive eating, 12–13
mood states, 67
Movement—Feel the Difference principle, 10, 138–149
    benefits of and barriers to movement, 145–147
    closing sessions, 148
    compensatory, compulsive, and over-exercise, 147–148
    considerations and adaptations, 140
    exercise versus movement, 141–142
    intuitive movement, 142–144
    session aim, 139
    between-session exercises, 141, 148

N
neurodivergent populations
    with disordered eating, 74
    fullness cues, 101
    gentle nutrition considerations with, 152
    interoceptive cues, 64
    setting movement goals, 147
normative discontent, 129
nutrition, 14–17. *see also* Honor Your Health—Gentle Nutrition principle
    challenging thought patterns session, 90
    dietary quality, 15–17
    eating behaviors, 14–15
    physical activity, 17

O
obesity, 51
obsessive thoughts, 77
open groups, 34
open weighing, 50
openness, encouraging, 49
opposite action, 133
oppression, weight-related, 57
orthorexia, 17, 22–23
OSFED (other specified feeding and eating disorders), 23–24
over-exercise, 147–148
overweight, 51

P

paired snack activity, 101, 109
parental coercive feeding strategies, 12
Pew Research Center, 135
physical activity, 17, 118–119. *see also* Movement—Feel the Difference principle
physical health, 18
The Picky Eater's Recovery Book (Thomas et al.), 25
play foods, 156–157
poverty, 89
principles of intuitive eating, 8–10
    Challenge the Food Police principle, 8–9, 87–98
    Cope with Your Emotions with Kindness principle, 9, 113–123
    Discover the Satisfaction Factor principle, 9, 99–112
    Feel Your Fullness principle, 9, 99–112
    Honor Your Health—Gentle Nutrition principle, 10, 150–165
    Honor Your Hunger principle, 8, 62–71
    introducing at sessions, 39
    Make Peace with Food principle, 8, 72–86
    Movement—Feel the Difference principle, 10, 138–149
    Reject Diet Culture principle, 8, 45–60
    Respect Your Body principle, 9–10, 124–137
problem-focused coping, 121
progress, celebrating, 166–174
    considerations and adaptations, 167
    exercises for, 168–170
    planning for future exercises, 170–171
    reflecting on program exercise, 172
    sample plan, 173–174
    session aim, 167
    between-session exercises, 168
protein, 108
psychological health, 13–14
psychological reactance theory, 31–32
public policies, 156

R

Recovery Record app, 26
RED-S (relative energy deficiency in sport), 28
reframing thoughts
    body appreciation, 131
    cognitive defusion and, 102
    food-related beliefs, 93
    junk foods, 157
    self-compassion, 55
Reject Diet Culture principle, 8, 45–60
    acknowledging weight, 49–52
    closing session, 60
    considerations and adaptations, 47–48
    costs of micromanaging eating, 56–59
    diets defined, 46, 52–53
    encouraging openness and curiosity, 49
    expectations of session, 46–47
    identifying problem with diets, 53–54
    nurturing self-compassion, 54–55
    session aim, 46
    between-session exercises, 59–60
relative energy deficiency in sport (RED-S), 28
Resch, Elyse, 7
research, 13–18
    health behaviors and nutrition, 14–17
    physical health, 18
    psychological health, 13–14
Respect Your Body principle, 9–10, 124–137
    closing sessions, 136
    considerations and adaptations, 125–126
    cultivating body respect, 130–133
    life without body negativity, 129–130
    overview, 127–129
    responding to body talk, 133–135
    session aim, 125
    between-session exercises, 126–127, 136
    social media, 135
restrictive eating, 22–23, 51. *see also* ARFID
    early satiety after, 100
    increased attentional biases with, 128
role-play exercises
    arguing for intuitive movement, 147
    Body Project, 32
    dieting dissonance, 54
    food-related conversations and comments, 94–96
    habituation dissonance, 82–83
    reframing with self-compassionate thoughts, 55

responding to body talk, 134–135

S

satisfaction, 9. *see also* Discover the Satisfaction Factor principle
self-care
    challenges with, 76
    checking in on, 117–118
    disrupting interoceptive awareness, 106
    overview, 69–70
self-compassion, 54–55, 160–162
self-criticism, 160
self-harm, 76
self-induced vomiting, 22–23
self-monitoring, 131–132
self-objectification, 12
self-weighing, 50, 51–52, 131–132
Sensory Considerations worksheet, 110, 116
shame
    associating hunger with, 63
    diet culture evoking, 8
    emotional eating, 116
    fears of fullness, 106
    longer-term implications of, 159–160
    medical conditions engendering, 27
    nurturing self-compassion, 54
    self-weighing, 50, 51
    values pie chart and, 59
shortening treatment
    eight sessions, 42
    four sessions, 41
    six sessions, 42
significant others, involving, 36
single-led groups, 34
sleep, 146
SMART goals, 40
snack pairings, 101, 109, 116
social comparison theory, 32
social comparisons, 75, 89
social media
    body image concerns and, 135
    fitness advertisements on, 147
social pressure, 107
social support, 12
Spain, Emily, 17

stereotypes, 19–20
stigma, 19–20, 35, 57, 134
stress, 69, 117
systematic desensitization, 83

T

target weights, 24
telehealth, 36
ten principles of intuitive eating, 8–10, 11, 15, 17
theoretical framework, 31–32
    acceptance model, 31
    cognitive dissonance theory, 32
    social comparison theory, 32
    theory of psychological reactance, 31–32
thin ideal, 21, 32
Thomas, Jennifer, 25
thought defusion, 9
timing, meal, 107–108
trauma, 29, 123
trauma-informed approaches, 29
Tribole, Evelyn, 7
27-item intuitive eating scale, 13

U

ultra-processed foods, 156
unconditional permission to eat, 16
upward comparisons, 32
urge surfing, 121–122

V

values pie chart, 58–59
vegetables, 128
virtual treatment, 36

W

weight, acknowledging, 49–52
weight restoration
    determining if clients are ready, 24–25, 49
    habituation fears, 84
weight science, 127–128
wellness trends, 8, 22, 46, 54–55, 78
women of color, 21
writing exercises, 131, 141

Y

yo-yo dieting, 22

Real change *is* possible

For more than forty-five years, New Harbinger has published proven-effective self-help books and pioneering workbooks to help readers of all ages and backgrounds improve mental health and well-being, and achieve lasting personal growth. In addition, our spirituality books offer profound guidance for deepening awareness and cultivating healing, self-discovery, and fulfillment.

Founded by psychologist Matthew McKay and Patrick Fanning, New Harbinger is proud to be an independent, employee-owned company. Our books reflect our core values of integrity, innovation, commitment, sustainability, compassion, and trust. Written by leaders in the field and recommended by therapists worldwide, New Harbinger books are practical, accessible, and provide real tools for real change.

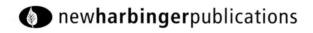

MORE BOOKS from NEW HARBINGER PUBLICATIONS

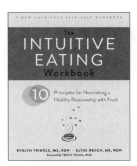

THE INTUITIVE EATING WORKBOOK

Ten Principles for Nourishing a Healthy Relationship with Food

978-1626256224 / US $25.95

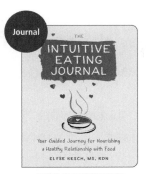

THE INTUITIVE EATING JOURNAL

Your Guided Journey for Nourishing a Healthy Relationship with Food

978-1684037087 / US $18.95

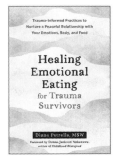

HEALING EMOTIONAL EATING FOR TRAUMA SURVIVORS

Trauma-Informed Practices to Nurture a Peaceful Relationship with Your Emotions, Body, and Food

978-1648481178 / US $19.95

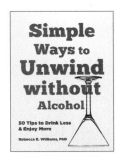

SIMPLE WAYS TO UNWIND WITHOUT ALCOHOL

50 Tips to Drink Less and Enjoy More

978-1648482342 / US $18.95

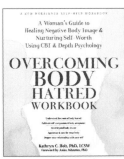

OVERCOMING BODY HATRED WORKBOOK

A Woman's Guide to Healing Negative Body Image and Nurturing Self-Worth Using CBT and Depth Psychology

978-1648482076 / US $26.95

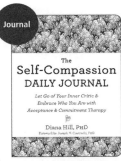

THE SELF-COMPASSION DAILY JOURNAL

Let Go of Your Inner Critic and Embrace Who You Are with Acceptance and Commitment Therapy

978-1648482496 / US $18.95

newharbingerpublications

1-800-748-6273 / newharbinger.com

(VISA, MC, AMEX / prices subject to change without notice)

Follow Us

QUICK TIPS for THERAPISTS

Written by leading clinicians, Quick Tips for Therapists are free e-mails, sent twice a month, to help enhance your client sessions.

Visit **newharbinger.com/quicktips** to sign up today!

Did you know there are **free tools** you can download for this book?

Free tools are things like **worksheets**, **guided meditation exercises**, and **more** that will help you get the most out of your book.

You can download free tools for this book—whether you bought or borrowed it, in any format, from any source—from the New Harbinger website. All you need is a NewHarbinger.com account. Just use the URL provided in this book to view the free tools that are available for it. Then, click on the "download" button for the free tool you want, and follow the prompts that appear to log in to your NewHarbinger.com account and download the material.

You can also save the free tools for this book to your **Free Tools Library** so you can access them again anytime, just by logging in to your account! Just look for this button on the book's free tools page.

+ Save this to my free tools library

If you need help accessing or downloading free tools, visit **newharbinger.com/faq** or contact us at customerservice@newharbinger.com.